STUDENT NOTES

Epidemiology in Medical Practice

D. J. P. Barker BSc, MD, PhD, FRCP, FFCM
Director and Professor of Clinical Epidemiology, Medical Research Council
Environmental Epidemiology Unit, University of
Southampton; Honorary Consultant Physician, Royal South
Hants Hospital, Southampton, UK

G. Rose MA, DM, DSc, FRCP, FFCM, FRCGP
Professor of Epidemiology, London School of Hygiene and
Tropical Medicine; Honorary Consultant Physician, St Mary's
Hospital, London, UK

FOURTH EDITION

CHURCHILL LIVINGSTONE
EDINBURGH LONDON MELBOURNE AND NEW YORK 1990

CHURCHILL LIVINGSTONE
Medical Division of Pearson Professional Ltd

Distributed in the United States of America by
Churchill Livingstone Inc., 650 Avenue of the Americas,
New York. N.Y. 10011, and by associated companies,
branches and representatives throughout the world.

© Longman Group Limited 1976, 1979, 1984
© Longman Group UK Limited 1990

First edition 1976
Second edition 1979
Third edition 1984
Reprinted 1987
Fourth edition 1990
    Reprinted 1992
    Reprinted 1994
    Reprinted 1995

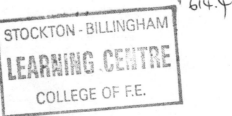
ISBN 0-443-03783-3

British Library Cataloguing in Publication Data
A catalogue record for this book is available from the British Library

Library of Congress Cataloging in Publication Data
A catalog record is available from the Library of Congress

The
publisher's
policy is to use
paper manufactured
from sustainable forests

Produced by Longman Singapore Publishers (Pte) Ltd.
Printed in Singapore

Epidemiology in Medical Practice

This book is to be returned
the l

Preface

Epidemiology, the study of the distribution and determinants of disease in human populations, has always been an integral part of medical practice. The geographical distribution of a disease, the variations in its frequency at different times, and the special characteristics of people affected by it, are part of the basic description by means of which it is defined and recognized. In times when medical practice was overshadowed by epidemics, doctors were inevitably concerned with disease distributions, and this concern must have been heightened by early successes, such as that with cholera, whereby study of the distributions led to identification of causes and thence to prevention.

In the last few decades the methods of epidemiology have been explored and refined, and attention has expanded from acute infectious and dietary diseases to the chronic degenerative disorders that are now the principal causes of death and disability in industrialized societies. To solve some problems related to prevention and control, and to evaluate certain aspects of health services, large and prolonged investigations have proved necessary: to meet this need, the full-time epidemiologist has emerged. However, clinicians will always have a central role in epidemiology.

This book is intended for clinicians and medical undergraduates. The first section introduces the methods used to describe diseases in populations. Measurement of the frequency and changing patterns of diseases is essential to ensure that the deployment of medical resources matches the community's needs. Without such measurements, needs for health care and prevention may be unidentified and unmet. The second section describes the application of epidemiology in the discovery of causes of disease. Most hypotheses about causation subsequently confirmed by epidemiological methods have arisen from the day-to-day experience of alert clinicians, and many more will do so in the future. In the past, doctors tended to regard the practical application of these discoveries to the prevention of disease as being outside their sphere of responsibility. However, in obstetrics, paediatrics and general practice, prevention has become accepted as a normal part of medical practice, and concern for disease prevention is gaining ground in other branches of medicine. In the third section an account is given of four aspects of patient care which require an understanding of epidemiology: screening, prognosis, epidemics, and the evaluation of medical services.

Southampton and London, 1990   D.J.P.B.
                                                                  G.R.

Contents

Description of disease in the community

1. Community diagnosis

Decisions on the management of a patient require a clinical diagnosis, based on the history, examination and special investigations. Management of ill-health in the community as a whole requires a community diagnosis which rests on epidemiological information. A community diagnosis can be expressed in terms of *rates* which relate data on illness to data on the whole population. No single set of statistics describes the illness in a community, and our picture of the frequency and causes of illness is built up from studying the various ways in which disease alters people's life expectancy and behaviour. *Mortality* data are widely used because of their ready availability, certification of death being a legal requirement in many countries; but unless a disease is usually fatal, data on *morbidity* (the frequency of illness) are preferable, although often difficult to obtain.

This chapter illustrates how epidemiology may be used to diagnose national and local problems, to show changing patterns of disease and to reveal the existence of groups of people within the community who are at special risk. The sources of epidemiological information are either routinely collected health statistics, for example death certificates or hospital discharges, or the results of special surveys. Chapter 2 describes the kinds of population, mortality and morbidity statistics that are freely available in many industrialized countries. Chapter 3 describes the techniques used in special surveys. In this first chapter some examples of disease rates are given. The derivation and use of rates is discussed in detail in Chapter 4.

National problems

For most of humankind, low living standards are the dominant influence determining ill-health and death. One sensitive

Table 1.1 Infant mortality rates for selected countries (1986)

Country	Infant deaths per 1000 live births
Argentina	35
Yugoslavia	27
USSR	25
Cuba	14
USA	10
England and Wales	9
Netherlands	8
Sweden	6
Japan	5

indicator of a low standard of living is provided by the *infant mortality rate* (the number of children under one year old dying during a year related to the number of live births in the same year). Table 1.1 gives some examples, and shows how large the range is.

In most industrialized countries today the proportion of deaths ascribed to infection is less than 1%, their former place as the major cause of death having been taken by cardiovascular disease, cerebrovascular disease, neoplasms and chronic bronchitis. Coincidentally with the decline in infectious disease and the consequent fall in mortality during the past century there has been an upsurge in the frequency of a group of diseases, including coronary heart disease, appendicitis, colonic diverticulosis — diseases associated with affluence, or the so-called 'diseases of industrialization'. Thus improvements in standards of living bring losses to health as well as gains.

International mortality comparisons identify special national problems such as alcoholic cirrhosis in France, hypertension and stroke in Eastern Europe, and coronary heart disease in Finland and Scotland. Studies of people who have migrated from a country with high mortality from a particular disease to one with lower mortality, or vice versa, are of particular interest. Migrants tend to acquire the disease pattern of their host country. For example, the Japanese in America have much lower rates for stroke than in their homeland, whereas the risk of coronary heart disease among migrants from southern Italy to Australia increases after some years in their new country to approach that of the native-born Australian.

Similar findings have come from international studies of blood pressure, diabetes and hyperuricaemia. Among the Polynesian inhabitants of certain Pacific islands there is little or no tendency for blood pressure to rise with age; diabetes is uncommon; and blood urate levels are low. These distinctive features are lost in Polynesian communities that have migrated to New Zealand. Evidently the industrialized country's environment has an adverse effect on hypertension, diabetes and gout. International differences in the frequency of disease seem mainly to reflect the influence of environment and way of life rather than of a distinctive genetic constitution — a satisfactory conclusion from the viewpoint of preventive medicine. Genetic influences, for example on blood pressure, are more important in determining differences between individuals.

Regional problems

During the second half of the last century the annual analyses of death certificates carried out by the Registrar General showed consistently higher death rates in the northern and western regions of England and Wales than in the South and East. Most of the deaths were due to infectious diseases, and inequalities in living standards — hygiene, housing, diet — were the major contributory factors in the inequality of mortality. Remarkably, the decline in mortality during this century has not eliminated the disparity between regions and social classes. Table 1.2 presents data from the regions of England and Wales in 1985, with

Table 1.2 Regional variations in mortality in England and Wales in 1985

Region	Standardized mortality ratios	
	Men	Women
North-west	112	111
North	113	112
Wales	105	103
Yorks and Humberside	106	103
W. Midlands	105	103
E. Midlands	100	100
South-west	89	92
South-east	93	94
E. Anglia	90	94
England and Wales	100	100

all-causes mortality expressed as standardized mortality ratios. These ratios, which are described in detail on page 54, are calculated so that the overall ratio for England and Wales is 100. Regions with ratios above 100 have above average mortality rates, after allowance for the age structure of their populations, and vice versa.

Information about mortality is easier to obtain than information about morbidity, since the law requires that the occurrence of every death and its cause are recorded on a death certificate. No such legal dictates apply to the occurrence of non-fatal illness. Nevertheless, morbidity surveys carried out during the past century, such as the British Medical Association's extensive 1889 survey of rickets, rheumatism, chorea, cancer and urinary calculus, have revealed marked regional variations. Today such variations are seen in a range of common and important diseases, including coronary heart disease, peptic ulcer, gallstones and diabetes. They are seen also in children's diseases, such as anencephaly and Perthes' disease of the hip. This implies that the variation of disease within Britain is not just a dwindling legacy of past inequalities but in part at least is due to influences that are still present.

Socio-economic influences, definable only in general terms such as income and population density, are to some extent implicated in the regional variation in mortality and morbidity; and so too, to a lesser extent, are adverse effects of urban life, occupational factors and, possibly, genetic factors. Differences in medical care play little part and most of the variation remains unexplained. The existence of these geographical variations within industrialized countries such as Britain offers tantalizing clues to the causation of disease. And the discovery of modifiable influences in the environment which adversely affect the health of people living in certain parts of a country is a major challenge to preventive medicine.

Time trends

During this century some diseases have increased in frequency (for example, ischaemic heart disease), some have decreased (the infections), and some have risen and declined (for example, appendicitis). Acquired immunodeficiency syndrome (AIDS) appeared abruptly in the USA in 1981. Duodenal ulcer was first described at the beginning of the century, reached a peak frequency in the mid-1950s, and is now becoming less common. The frequency of

Table 1.3 Some conditions for which mortality rates have risen (England and Wales)

Cause of death	% increase 1975–85	
	Men	Women
Diabetes mellitus	55	38
Cirrhosis of liver	50	31
Prostate cancer	47	—
Oesophageal cancer	42	22
Skin cancers	36	16
Osteomyelitis	33	46
Multiple sclerosis	17	20
Lung cancer	(−2)	42

renal stones has risen steeply in Europe since the turn of the century (in Norway, for example, there was a 200% increase in hospital admissions between 1920 and 1960). Interestingly the increase, although steep, has not been continuous. In Europe a transient decline was noted during and after both world wars, and in Japan a similarly transient decline followed the Second World War. Thus whatever the influences that have given rise to the increase, they were checked during the adverse condition of war. The fluctuation in incidence of so many common diseases reflects the rapid changes in environment and way of life that have characterized this century. It suggests that the causes are modifiable and hence that their identification could lead to prevention.

Some illustrations of diseases whose mortality rates (numbers of deaths related to population size) have shown an alarming recent rise are given in Table 1.3. Changes of this kind, recorded by routine statistics, must be regarded as an alarm signal calling urgently for further enquiry. For example, deaths from bronchial asthma among young people in Britain have increased recently, when therapeutic advances should have led to a fall. It is essential to discover whether this is due to misuse of treatment or to a rising incidence; and if the latter, which allergies are involved.

Often the first clue to a new problem comes from astute clinicians, as happened when gastrointestinal haemorrhage was noticed in association with non-steroidal anti-inflammatory drugs.

High-risk groups

Even within one area and at one particular time the frequency of disease can be highly variable. For example, in Britain tuberculosis has virtually disappeared among young well-housed white people but remains prevalent among immigrants, especially those from Asia. All the major killing diseases are now associated with a low socio-economic level, and this is reflected in the all-causes mortality gradients. At present, all-causes mortality in unskilled labourers and their wives is almost twice as high as among professional families, so that classification by occupation identifies a group with special risk for most major disorders — not only infections, but cardiovascular diseases, bronchitis, peptic ulcer, cirrhosis and a number of cancers. This is relevant not only to aetiology and prevention but also to the provision of medical services such as screening.

Table 1.4 illustrates how the broad indication of a problem given by routine statistics can be narrowed down by progressive enquiry until finally a sufficiently high-risk group has been delineated to call for effective action. A series of simple assessments finally identifies a group of men — all smokers with hypertension and abnormal ECG — in whom risk of death from coronary heart disease is four times greater than average.

Mortality statistics may identify occupational risks. For example, widespread use of chemicals in industry can involve unforeseeable health hazards, such as coronary heart disease in rayon manufacturers exposed to carbon disulphide, or haemangiosarcoma of the liver in vinyl chloride workers. Mortality is not an adequate or early indicator of risk, and there is a strong case for a system of routine morbidity statistics, at least among workers exposed to chemicals. A comparable monitoring system for drug toxicity in patients is provided by the Committee on Safety of Medicines.

Table 1.4 Coronary heart disease mortality rates in middle-aged men in London

Group	% dying of CHD in 15 years
All men	7
All smokers	9
All smokers with hypertension	17
All smokers with hypertension and abnormal ECG	28

Systems are being developed to monitor health in the locality of industrial sources of pollution, such as nuclear installations.

Defining priorities

Medical resources are and always will be insufficient, in terms of both money and skills, to meet demands for them (see Ch. 10). To determine their best use is a complex matter, but one consideration is the priority due to those diseases that impose the greatest burden on the community. Unfortunately this burden cannot be adequately expressed in any one form. Ultimately for each major condition we need separate measures of (1) mortality, (2) symptomatic burden, and (3) disability. The first of these is now reasonably well documented, but detailed or complete assessments of the other two will require special surveys and improvements in routine statistics. As an indirect guide to symptomatic burden one may look at numbers of hospital admissions and general practice consultation rates; sickness absence data provide some measure of disability.

Table 1.5 takes each of these four ways of measuring the community burden, and for each measure it lists in order the five leading contributors in England and Wales. The variation in these lists shows the importance of not confining attention to any one simple measure of the priority due to different diseases. For example, the most frequent causes of hospital admission tend to be acute illnesses, whereas chronic conditions impose much larger burdens in terms of bed occupancy: even today patients with mental illness or handicap occupy 38% of all hospital beds in the country. It is worth noting also that accidents or poisoning feature in the 'top-five' for each measure of community burden.

Unfortunately, doctors tend to regard common disorders as less interesting and as a result these disorders often do not get the priority they deserve. Such information as that set out in Table 1.5 can help to give a sense of proportion to teaching and to the planning of services and research. The commonest conditions are likely to be those in which medical advance will benefit the most people.

Table 1.5 The five leading diagnoses, in rank order, according to each of various measures of frequency (England and Wales)

| Mortality | | Hospital admissions | GP consultations | | Certified sickness absence from work (days lost, men) |
Males	Females		Males	Females	
Coronary heart disease	Coronary heart disease	Cancers	Injuries	Mental disorder	Mental disorder
Stroke	Stroke	Coronary heart disease	Upper respiratory tract infection	Upper respiratory tract infection	Cardiovascular disorder
Lung cancer	Breast cancer	Mental disorder	Mental disorder	Injuries	Arthritis
Accidents/poisoning	Lung cancer	Hernia	Hypertension	Hypertension	Injuries
Bronchitis/emphysema	Accidents/poisoning	Poisoning	Bronchitis	Bronchitis	Bronchitis/emphysema/asthma

2. Sources of information: routine statistics

In this chapter a brief description is given of the kinds of population, mortality and morbidity statistics that are freely available in many industrialized countries. Although the examples quoted are generally based on statistics from Britain, there are principles in the sources of data and causes of error that are common to all routine statistics.

Population statistics

In many countries a population census is carried out every 10 years at around the beginning of the decade. Data are collected about the geographical and economic characteristics of the population, and the characteristics of individuals and households. Only certain of these data are commonly used for the denominator in routine health statistics since medical records, which usually provide the numerator in the calculation of rates, contain only limited social, economic and geographical information.

The population of England was first estimated in 1086 from the numbers of families recorded in the Domesday Book, and then in 1695 from a count of the number of hearths. Since 1801 there have been full decennial censuses. The reconstruction of the country's population growth which these data allow (Fig. 2.1) is of considerable medical interest, showing as it does the way in which growth accompanied the agricultural and industrial revolutions and antedated the major advances in medical care.

Since 1838 there has been in England and Wales an enforced system of registration of births and deaths. It is therefore possible to study in detail the changes in birth rates and death rates (annual numbers of births and deaths per thousand population) that have underlain the increases in the population. The death rate declined sharply after 1870, largely as a result of the reduced mortality from

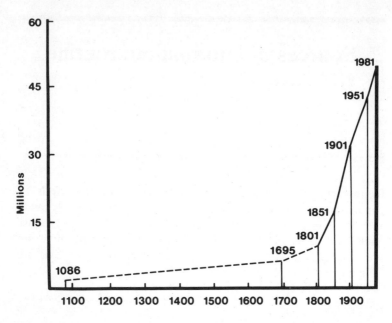

Fig. 2.1 Population growth in England and Wales.

infectious diseases which followed improvements in hygiene and the general standards of living. Although the birth rate also declined from around 1880 onwards it remained in excess of the death rate, and the rise in population therefore continued. Subtraction of the death rate from the birth rate gives the current annual growth rate of a population (exclusive of migration). Some European countries have now reached zero or even negative growth rates. Elsewhere are countries such as Syria, Kuwait and Iraq where the rates exceed 3.5%, at which level the size of the population is doubled in less than 20 years.

The basic unit of a census is the enumeration district, which comprises a small number of households. Error rates in censuses vary markedly between non-industrialized countries, where censuses are often carried out in the face of formidable practical difficulties, and industrialized countries, where censuses provide some of the most accurate of all routine statistics. Two kinds of error that are known to occur readily are the omission of very young children and inaccurate recording of age — especially in countries where birth registration is not effective.

Mortality statistics

Data on the numbers and causes of deaths in the United Kingdom have been published by the Registrar General since 1839. These data derive from death certificates, issued usually by the doctor at the time of death. Table 2.1 shows common certified causes of death in England and Wales during 1985. The finding that 31% of deaths in men were ascribed to coronary heart disease and 9% to cerebrovascular disease may, in part, reflect current fashions in diagnosis, especially of those elderly patients in whom extensive investigation is not warranted. (In the last century fashion permitted deaths to be ascribed to 'privation' and 'despair'; and deaths from 'teething' were recorded as late as 1920.) Nevertheless the data are important: they reveal, for example, the immense economic importance of accidents and suicide, which kill a disproportionate number of younger adults — 34% of deaths in men under the age of 45 years, and 17% in women aged under 45.

The internationally agreed form of death certificate has two parts. The doctor records in Part 1 the disorders leading directly to death and, in Part 2, other disorders that may have contributed to death but are unrelated to those in Part 1. Further data are supplied by a relative or friend who takes the completed death certificate to the registrar of deaths and is asked for personal details of the deceased, including occupation and place and date of birth.

Table 2.1 Common certified causes of death (England and Wales, 1985)

Condition	% all deaths	% deaths under 45 years	% deaths 45 years and over
Men			
Coronary heart disease	31	9	33
Neoplasms	25	14	26
Cerebrovascular disease	9	3	10
Pneumonia and influenza	4	2	4
Accidents and suicide	4	34	2
Chronic bronchitis	3	0.1	3
Women			
Coronary heart disease	24	2	25
Neoplasms	23	29	22
Cerebrovascular disease	15	4	16
Pneumonia and influenza	6	2	6
Accidents and suicide	3	17	2
Chronic bronchitis	1	0.1	1

If a death certificate states that further information about the cause of death may become available at a later date (for example following post-mortem examination) the registrar sends the certifying doctor a form on which the additional information may be recorded. The coroner informs the registrar about deaths reported to him.

The completed record on each death in England and Wales is sent to the *Office of Population Censuses and Surveys* (OPCS) where the underlying cause of death is coded according to the *International Classification of Disease*. This classification, which is published by the World Health Organization, was originally designed to classify causes of death, but was later expanded to cover causes of morbidity. It has been repeatedly revised to meet statistical and medical needs. From the coded data annual statistical reviews are published by the Registrar General. (These and other publications referred to in this chapter are detailed in the reference list at the end.)

The OPCS does not make a routine check on the accuracy of mortality data, and in their interpretation possible sources of error must be considered. Errors may occur in the completion of death certificates, through incorrect diagnosis of the cause of death and through errors and omissions when the causes of death are written down. Studies of a number of diseases have shown that the accuracy of death certification decreases with advancing age of the deceased. The usefulness of death certificates for epidemiology depends on the particular disease. For example, whereas deaths certified as resulting from motor neurone disease give a reliable picture of the distribution of the disease, those certified as due to dementia reflect only the distribution of mental hospitals. Seemingly for most people with dementia who die outside hospital some other underlying cause of death is recorded.

It is a feature of epidemiology that where, as often happens, errors tend to cancel each other out, data may be of value for population studies although too unreliable for use in individual cases. In one study the ante-mortem and autopsy diagnoses were compared in 9501 hospital deaths occurring in 75 hospitals. The overall frequency of a number of diseases was similar in the ante-mortem and post-mortem diagnoses, despite many disagreements in individual patients. For example, clinical diagnoses of carcinoma of the rectum were confirmed at autopsy in only 67% of cases, but the incorrect clinical diagnoses were balanced by an almost identical number of lesions diagnosed for the first time at autopsy.

For certain years the Registrar General (England and Wales) coded all causes of death given on certificates rather than the underlying cause alone. These data allow examination of disorders, such as Paget's disease of bone, which though often present at the time of death are not usually recorded as the underlying cause. They are also free from those errors that arise when either the certifying doctor incorrectly selects one cause of death as the underlying one, or when there are several coincident pathological conditions from which selection of one as the underlying condition is more or less arbitrary.

Occupational mortality

Recording of occupation on death registration forms allows the numbers of deaths occurring among people in any occupation to be related to the total number of people known from population census data to be employed in this way. It is well known that occupations such as coal-mining are associated with an above average mortality. But mortality in an occupational group reflects both the specific hazards of the occupation and the social conditions with which it is associated. Not only the coal-miners themselves but their wives also have a high mortality, which points to adverse influences in the neighbourhood of coal-mines, such as bad housing.

The Registrar General publishes analyses on occupational mortality approximately every 10 years. Difficulties in interpretation of the data arise because the numerator and denominator used to calculate the rates are not strictly comparable. The numerator derives from a description of occupation recorded at the time of death by a relative or some other person. The denominator derives from information given by the head of the household about his or her occupation and that of other people in the house at the time of the census. A person's occupation may be coded differently from a description given while they are alive than from one given after their death. Another source of error arises when people change occupation, for they will be included in the rates for their final occupation only. The OPCS does not make routine checks on the accuracy of occupational data recorded on death certificates or during censuses, but surveys have demonstrated major errors in upwards of 10% of all records.

Morbidity statistics

Data on morbidity are less readily obtained than data on mortality. However, in most countries of the world some insight into morbidity can be gained from two sources, hospital inpatient data and notifications of disease. Additional sources that may be used in some countries include other parts of the medical care system, notably general practice, and the social security records. In this section the sources most widely used in Britain are described in some detail: others are listed at the end.

Hospital inpatient statistics

Patients' clinical records at the time of discharge form the basis of hospital inpatient statistics, whose primary purpose is to assist planning of hospital services. As indicators of morbidity in the community, hospital records have the merit of diagnostic accuracy but the great disadvantage of being unrepresentative. Hospitals are preoccupied only with certain types of illnesses, such as those requiring surgery or emergency treatment.

It is natural for doctors to be interested in statistical reviews of the patients they themselves are treating, and during the past two centuries there have been many studies of the frequency of different causes of hospital admission. For example, in 1874 a Norwich surgeon wrote to other surgeons in the large hospitals throughout Britain and obtained from each the number of cases of bladder stone treated in the previous 5 years as a proportion of all inpatients. The results confirmed the general impression among Norfolk doctors that bladder˙ stones were exceptionally common in their county; and the possible causes of this were the subject of intense and diverse speculation.

Figure 2.2 shows the varying discharge rates following cholecystectomy in the hospital regions of England and Wales. The rates range from 5.5 per 10 000 population in the North-West Thames region to 9.5 per 10 000 in Wales. This variation could be due mainly to differences in surgical practice. However, a study of the autopsy prevalence of gallstones in nine towns showed that prevalences were closely related to cholecystectomy rates. It seems therefore that Figure 2.2 reveals a real geographical variation in gallstone disease and reflects the causation of this common disease.

Acute appendicitis is another common disease for which

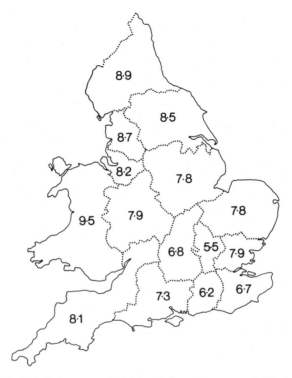

Fig. 2.2   Hospital discharge rates following cholecystectomy per 10 000 population in England and Wales (HIPE data) 1981

hospital statistics have revealed geographical differences in frequency within Britain. Hospital discharge rates following appendicectomy for acute appendicitis are higher in Ireland, Scotland, Wales and northern England than in southern England. One difficulty in interpreting this variation is that a proportion of removed appendices are found to be normal, yet in some of these cases the diagnosis of appendicitis still appears on hospital records. Hospital discharge rates therefore overestimate the incidence of acute appendicitis, and variations among areas may reflect different recording practices and surgical policies as well as true variations in incidence. However, surveys in Britain and Ireland have shown that the percentage of removed appendices that do not show pathological changes does not vary greatly from place to place, being around 30%. Hence differences in hospital discharge rates may be used to examine differences in the frequency of acute appendicitis. These differences have been shown to relate closely to differences in housing and hygiene, and support other evidence suggesting that appendicitis is primarily related to improved 'Western' hygiene.

Hospital Inpatient Enquiry. With the inception of the National Health Service it was readily recognized that there was the opportunity to create a comprehensive national scheme for recording information about hospital admissions. Such a scheme would give data on the variations of morbidity within the community, and on the utilization of hospital services by different groups of people. The Hospital Inpatient Enquiry (HIPE) was instituted and since 1958 has required detailed information on every tenth discharge from (or death in) all NHS hospitals in England and Wales, other than psychiatric ones. In Scotland, since 1961 the Scottish Home and Health Department has collected data on all non-obstetric discharges.

Collection of HIPE data depends upon completion of a standard form for every tenth patient discharged. Identification, administrative and clinical data are transcribed from the patient's notes. The administrative data include the date the patient was put on the waiting list, the source and date of admission, the speciality, the date of discharge or death, and the destination on discharge or transfer. The clinical data include the principal condition causing admission, other relevant conditions and the description and date of any operations performed. Completed forms are processed within the OPCS and analyses of the data are published annually.

There are two main features of HIPE data that limit their usefulness as indicators of morbidity in the community. Firstly, there is much variation from one disease to another in the proportion of patients who receive inpatient treatment. Secondly, the data are a sample of discharges and not a sample of patients. The Oxford Record Linkage study found that 16% of patients were admitted more than once in a year. Obviously a hospital discharge rate for a disease is compounded of the number of patients with the disease and the number of times each patient is admitted during a specified period. Since HIPE data do not allow the admissions of one patient to be linked together, the number of patients cannot be determined for any except non-recurrent illnesses.

The use of HIPE data is also limited by the nature and accuracy of the information recorded. There are, for example, no data on outpatient attendances, on severity of the disease, or on outcome other than death. Although the data can be used to study certain administrative problems such as local needs for maternity beds, figures on lengths of stay in hospital and numbers of operations performed are too crude an index of usage of hospital facilities for many purposes. Such information as is available suggests that the data recorded on principle diagnosis and operations are generally accurate, but for the second and third diagnoses accuracy is less.

The limitations of HIPE data sometimes lead doctors to dismiss them entirely as indicators of disease frequency. However, as the findings for gallstones and acute appendicitis suggest, this is too superficial a view. A recent survey recorded the frequency of Perthes' disease of the hip in three regions of England. HIPE data would be predicted to be an inappropriate indicator of the frequency of this disease, for many patients receive only outpatient treatment while others are repeatedly readmitted. Nevertheless the survey, which depended on direct notification of all new cases whether treated as in- or outpatients, confirmed the suggestion from HIPE analyses of higher rates in the north-west of England than in the south. Such results show that, used critically and with awareness of their limitations, hospital discharge data are a useful epidemiological tool.

Hospital Activity Analysis. Within a hospital each unit or department can more readily maintain its effectiveness if it has rapid feedback of information about its performance. HIPE does not meet this kind of short-term planning need and for this reason the Hospital Activity Analysis (HAA) was initiated in 1965. The data collected are mostly identical with those collected for HIPE, but HAA forms are completed for 100% of discharges and deaths. The forms are sent to the Regional Health Authority, where they are processed; analyses of numbers and types of patients treated, their lengths of stay, and the operations performed can be fed back to the consultants.

Since the HAA system collects information on all discharges, it is preferable to HIPE for studies of morbidity within one region. In order to collect HAA data for the whole of England and Wales it is necessary to apply separately to each of 15 health regions.

Inpatient statistics from the Mental Health Enquiry. The Mental Health Enquiry was begun in 1964 with the purpose of providing data on all psychiatric inpatients in England and Wales. Before this time the OPCS had collected data on admissions only from the main hospitals treating mental disorder. The Mental Health

Enquiry depends on completion of a form giving clinical and personal details of every patient admitted to psychiatric hospitals or units. The enquiry includes patients with mental illness, mental handicap and those in special hospitals such as Broadmoor. Information about patients permanently resident in institutions is obtained from periodic censuses.

Morbidity in general practice

Much information on morbidity is recorded by general practitioners in the course of their routine work, and general practice records reflect more closely the true relative frequencies of most diseases than do hospital or mortality records. Although the diagnostic information available in general practice is often less precise than in hospital, the data are free from many of the biases that arise from selective referral and admission of patients to hospital. In countries where general practitioners are responsible for a defined list of people, data on the numbers of consultations for different disorders are readily converted into morbidity rates. Common disorders may be studied using the records of one practice, or a group of neighbouring practices, but the study of less common disorders requires amalgamation of records from many practices.

In 1955–56 the Royal College of General Practitioners undertook a national morbidity survey by collecting records of the consultations taking place in over 100 practices during one year. A second survey was carried out in 1970–71 and a third in 1981–82. Table 2.2 shows the increase in patients consulting with asthma and gout

Table 2.2 Patients' consulting rates for asthma and gout, at all ages, in the three national morbidity surveys*

| Disease | Patients consulting per 1000 persons | | |
	1955–56	1970–71	1981–82
Asthma			
Male	8.9	10.6	20.0
Female	8.1	8.6	15.9
Gout			
Male	1.2	2.7	4.6
Female	0.4	0.6	1.0

* RCGP, OPCS, DHSS. Morbidity statistics from general practice. Third national study 1981–2. HMSO, London. Series MB5 no. 1.

over the period of the surveys. Such information would not otherwise be available since it does not often lead to either hospital admission or death.

Currently in Britain 56 practices serving some 400 000 people make regular weekly returns on the frequency of infectious diseases and acute respiratory illnesses, and monthly returns on important non-infectious diseases. The information on infections serves as a system of routine surveillance providing, for example, the main surveillance of rubella. The data on chronic diseases serve as an indicator of regional variations in morbidity and of time-trends.

Notifications

Health departments demand notification of the occurrence of certain diseases so that they may have early warning of epidemics and can take appropriate action. In all member countries of the WHO the *quarantinable diseases* (cholera, plague, yellow fever, typhus and relapsing fever) are notifiable. In addition many countries have their own lists of locally important diseases, usually infectious or parasitic, whose occurrence must be notified.

Infectious and parasitic diseases. In the UK there has been a statutory obligation for the notification of certain infectious diseases since 1889. The list of notifiable diseases is amended periodically and currently for England and Wales comprises 29 diseases. In addition some local authorities have declared other diseases notifiable in their areas. The completeness of notification varies for different diseases. Only a small proportion of cases of whooping cough are notified and there is considerable under-notification even of disorders such as acute pyogenic meningitis. Notification of diseases such as diphtheria, which are uncommon, is more complete.

Although the incompleteness of notifications makes them of little value as absolute measures of disease frequency, changes in the number of notifications of a disease can reflect real changes in frequency. Figure 2.3 shows the relation between notifications for whooping cough in England and Wales since 1940 and the uptake of immunization. The sharp decline in uptake following public concern about neurological complications of immunization led to a rise in whooping cough. The notifications give an important measure of this dangerous trend.

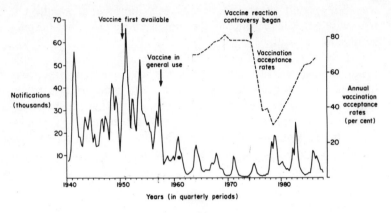

Fig. 2.3 Quarterly notifications of whooping cough in England and Wales 1940–87. (Source: Public Health Laboratory Service Communicable Disease Surveillance Centre.)

Congenital malformations. In 1961 accumulating evidence of the teratogenic effects of thalidomide led to its withdrawal from the market. During the 3 years when it was marketed in England and Wales at least 890 babies with gross limb malformations were born. In order that any future increase in frequency of a particular malformation should be detected early a national scheme for notification of congenital malformations was initiated in 1964. Local health authorities were asked to collect details of all malformed births by any means they chose, and each month to send the data on standard forms to the OPCS. The scheme is voluntary and data are collected in different ways in different areas, for example sometimes by the midwife or doctor attending the birth or sometimes by the health visitor during a follow-up visit. Not unexpectedly the completeness of ascertainment varies widely. A survey of anencephalic births showed that only a minority of areas recorded more than 90% of them, and reporting of less than 60% was by no means uncommon. Despite these shortcomings the registration scheme offers one method by which changes in the frequency of malformations may be detected. The influenza epidemics in England and Wales during 1966 and 1968 were followed by a 10% increase in reported cases of reduction deformities of the limbs and of cleft palate. This apparent relationship between influenza and the two malformations is also evident in the USA.

Registers

Whereas it is intended that notification of diseases should lead to immediate action to control outbreaks and epidemics, registration is intended to allow longer term observation and follow-up of patients. Many countries have registers for tuberculosis, for example.

In a number of industrialized countries *cancer registration* has recently been initiated. In Britain a national scheme for registration of all cases of malignant disease has operated since 1962. The routine recording of basic identification data on all cancer patients, together with the site and histological types of their lesions, is intended to provide information on the frequency of different forms of cancer, and on survival following diagnosis and treatment. Cancer registries facilitate studies of environmental hazards. From them population groups with high tumour incidences may be identified, for example rubber workers with bladder carcinoma and workers using mineral oil with scrotal carcinoma. Groups of people thought to be at risk from environmental hazards may be followed up, and the occurrence of carcinoma determined from the registers.

The responsibility for registration of patients with cancer rests with the hospital that treats them. Generally it is not doctors who carry out the registration but clerical staff, who abstract data from the clinical notes and send them on to the regional cancer registry, where national survey forms are completed and sent to the OPCS. Here computer processing results in a master file of patients, comprising personal, clinical and follow-up information.

Each cancer registry receives from the Registrar General photocopies of death certificates of patients in their area for whom malignant disease is given as a cause of death in either Part 1 or 2. This makes it possible for the registry to trace private patients and patients who die from malignant disease without attending hospital. Analyses of the national data are published periodically.

When interpreting data from cancer registries it is necessary to bear in mind that, unlike death certification, cancer registration is not a legal requirement. It is, therefore, not complete, and in a recent study of colonic cancer considerable under-registration was found in some registries. However, available evidence suggests that the accuracy of the description of diagnosis is high, with errors occurring in less than 1% of records.

In several city areas *coronary heart disease registers* have been set up in order to collate information recorded by hospitals, general practitioners and coroners' pathologists. The results have much enlarged our understanding of the natural history of this disease, particularly in regard to sudden death. It has been found, for example, that about two-thirds of all the deaths are medically unattended; perhaps this observation more than any other has made doctors aware of the importance of prevention.

Social security statistics

In industrialized countries the growth of social security systems has given an insight into the frequency with which different diseases result in absence from work as distinct from general practitioner consultation or hospital admission. In Britain a medical certificate is required before claims can be made for long-term sickness or injury benefit. On these certificates the diagnostic information is often rather general, since they are for the use of lay rather than medical staff, and sickness absence also reflects influences other than the type and severity of disease — for example job satisfaction. Nevertheless, the frequency of various certified causes of incapacity is of interest. Mental disorders, cardiovascular disease, arthritis injuries, chronic bronchitis and asthma emerge as the outstanding causes of lost working days in England and Wales (see Table 1.5, p.10). The ranking of diseases shown is strikingly different from the ranking of their contribution to mortality (Table 2.1) but is similar to the ranking of their contribution to general practitioner workload.

Other sources of morbidity data

In addition to the sources of morbidity data that have been described, other routine information is available about certain groups of people and diseases. It is impossible to itemize the many other sources of records that enterprising investigators can find in some areas, either in local government offices or in government departments, or in the files of charities and private organizations. However, for *young children* there are health visitor and child welfare clinic records which are collected and stored locally; for *schoolchildren* the school health service has records of routine examinations of schoolchildren, and of children in special schools; certain *industrial diseases* such as lead poisoning, chrome ulceration and epitheliomata due to tar, are notifiable to the

Chief Inspector of Factories and information on them is held by the Health and Safety Executive; and there are national registers of *disabled and blind* people.

Record linkage

Most of the sources of morbidity data that have been discussed give a picture of ill-health in terms of the number of events, such as admissions, attendances or periods off work, and not in terms of the number of sick people. To obtain data on the number of sick people it is necessary that the events relating to a single individual are linked together in some way. Linkage of records will give a picture of the full course of an illness and of the different illnesses occurring in the life of an individual. There is nothing new in the idea of record linkage and doctors have been carrying it out on a limited scale for decades, for example in tracing the birth records of children registered as handicapped to identify associations between obstetric events and subsequent physical and mental disorders. The coming of computers, however, has made record linkage feasible on a large scale and has brought visions of new kinds of medical information. A simple development will be the linkage of hospital discharges to readmissions and to mortality data so that badly needed, albeit crude, data on prognosis are obtained. Today coronary care units, with their expensive equipment and highly trained staff, do not usually know of the survival or death of their patients after discharge; there can be little disagreement that formal linkage of hospital and mortality records would be a major advance in coronary care. Beyond such simple uses of record linkage lie possibilities limited only by the resources available and the need to preserve the confidentiality of personal information. The linkage of general practitioner, outpatient and inpatient records would form the basis of a better understanding of the natural history of diseases such as hypertension. The subsequent medical histories of people exposed to drugs or industrial hazards would be readily available. Linkage of medical data with those of births and marriages would lead to an accumulating file of information on the familial occurrence of disease. Faced with an unconscious patient a clinician could use a linked record system to obtain immediate access to the complete medical history.

The basic requirements of a record linkage system are that each individual has a unique identification which labels all records relating to him or her, and that the system of record handling permits the records for each individual to be rapidly accessed, both for inspection of the data and for addition of new records. In Britain record linkage was pioneered in the Oxford study, but extension of this successful study to a national scheme is prevented by two factors. Firstly, the accumulation of medical, legal, social and other information on each individual on a single linked record represents to many people a threat to privacy that they cannot accept. Secondly, the financial and technical resources needed for a national scheme would be considerable. In the foreseeable future it seems likely that record linkage will be restricted to less controversial data, such as hospital discharges and causes of death, and to certain parts of the country only.

REFERENCES

This list gives some of the more widely used of the many publications related to UK and world health statistics. Most of the organizations responsible will make available data additional to those published.

Mortality and population statistics
Mortality statistics. England and Wales, OPCS, Series DH. Published annually in several parts by HMSO, London.
Annual Report of the Registrar General for Scotland. Published annually in two parts by HMSO, Edinburgh.
Annual Report of the Registrar General for Northern Ireland. Published annually by HMSO, Belfast.
World Health Statistics Annual. Vol. 1, *Vital Statistics and Causes of Death.* Published annually by WHO, Geneva.

Occupational mortality
Registrar General's Decennial Supplement England and Wales — Occupational Mortality Tables. Published decennially by HMSO, London.
Occupational Mortality. Published decennially by HMSO, Edinburgh.

Hospital inpatient statistics
Hospital Inpatient Enquiry, Main or Summary Tables. Published annually by HMSO, London.
Scottish Hospital Inpatient Statistics. Published annually by the Scottish Home and Health Department, Edinburgh.
Psychiatric Hospitals and Units in England and Wales; Inpatient Statistics from the Mental Health Enquiry. Published annually by HMSO, London, in the Statistical Research Report Series.

General practice
Morbidity Statistics from General Practice. The results of three national studies have been published by HMSO, London, in the *Studies on Medical and Population Subjects series.*

Notifications of infectious disease
Data published in the weekly and quarterly Returns of the Registrar Generals
for England and Wales, Scotland, and Northern Ireland.
Data also published in the Registrar General's annual publications, and in
Scottish Health Statistics published annually by HMSO, Edinburgh.

Congenital malformations
Data for England and Wales published as OPCS Series MB3.

Cancer
Registrar General's Statistical Review of England and Wales, Supplement on Cancer.
Published periodically by HMSO, London.
Cancer Registration 1965–67; Scottish Health Service Studies No. 26. Published in
1973 by the Scottish Home and Health Department, Edinburgh.

General health and social data
Social Trends. Published annually by Central Statistical Office, London.
Health and Personal Social Service Statistics for England. Published annually by
HMSO, London.

3. Sources of information: surveys

When describing disease in a community it is natural to turn first to data that are already available, that is, to routine statistics. Unfortunately, as has been shown in Chapter 2, information on many aspects of disease distribution cannot be obtained from a library. From a document such as a death certificate it is possible to learn about age, sex, residence and occupation, but not about more detailed social or physical characteristics. When these are important, as in many aetiological enquiries, or when morbidity or the natural history of disease needs to be assessed, it may be necessary to undertake a special survey.

Large surveys are complex and difficult undertakings that are not usually attempted without professional epidemiological and statistical help. But clinicians often have questions that can be answered by small-scale local surveys, and ideally all doctors ought to be competent to undertake such studies. This requires an awareness of the problems, and knowledge of some basic techniques.

Clinical case studies cannot answer epidemiological questions, since information is restricted to patients under medical care and this excludes on the one hand the numerous undiagnosed and milder cases, and on the other hand severer cases where death occurs outside hospital. More seriously, the results of a clinical case study provide numerators but not denominators, so that rates and risks cannot be calculated and differences between the sick and the healthy cannot be assessed. When, for example, the question was raised of whether non-steroidal anti-inflammatory agents lead to an increased risk of gastrointestinal haemorrhage, a survey of the treatment records of hospital cases of the disease could not provide the answer. It would be necessary to contrast the use of such drugs in patients with the disease with their use in the general population, matched for age, sex and other relevant factors.

Clinical studies, then, give detailed information about the characteristics of patients but these findings cannot be contrasted with those in other members of the same population who are free of the condition. On the other hand, epidemiological surveys tend to provide only rather superficial clinical information. In order to permit standardized examination of large numbers of people, mostly healthy, it may be necessary to accept lower standards of diagnostic accuracy and simpler types of investigation. As a consequence of this the problems of case definition and quality control of measurements tend to be considered more rigorously in population than in clinical studies.

Case definition

Clinical experience teaches us to think of a case of disease as being clearly defined, so that there is generally little problem in telling whether a particular patient has or has not got diseases such as diabetes or depression. This segregation of 'cases' and 'not cases' is substantially an artefact of the selective processes governing hospital admission. Hyperglycaemia or depression needs to be severe before it takes a patient to hospital, so that a hospital comprises two distinct subpopulations. One has high (symptomatic) levels, and the other resembles the general population. There is some overlap but it is not great. The same is true of many other personal characteristics associated with a risk of illness.

The situation in the community is quite different. Figure 3.1 shows the frequency distribution of depression scores in a community survey. The curve is continuous: 'normality' merges imperceptibly into 'clinical depression' (usually reckoned as requiring a score of 6+ on this scale). Moreover there is a graded increase in social disability across all levels of score, which suggests that the definition of 'a case of depression' is arbitrary not natural. Apart from a few inherited single-gene disorders such as Huntington's chorea it is hard to produce any convincing exceptions to the rule that in the general population disease behaves as a quantitative phenomenon. The question is not so much 'Has he got it?' as 'How much of it has he got?'

In clinical practice diagnosis is appropriate, but in population studies the ideal is rather to characterize the disease status of each

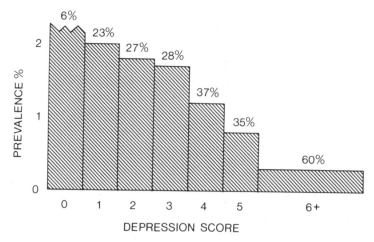

Fig. 3.1 Frequency distribution of depression scores in the general population: numbers above the bars are percentages of people at each score who require social support

individual quantitatively. Thus the results of a survey should generally be expressed by a distribution rather than by the frequency of 'disease', defined arbitrarily and very likely in different ways in different studies.

Even where it has been possible to measure disease quantitatively, there may be compelling practical reasons for defining what is thought to constitute 'a case'. Four distinct approaches are available:

1. *Statistical.* Following laboratory practice, 'abnormal' values can be defined as those lying two or more standard deviations away from the mean. This may be a helpful guide to the limits of what is common, but it carries no other medical significance, for it fixes the frequency of 'abnormal' values of everything at around 5%.

2. *Clinical.* This defines abnormality in terms of current state of health. For example, individuals are more likely to have symptoms if their blood pressure is above a certain level, and this level defines their liability to be recognized as clinical cases.

3. *Prognostic.* In a 50-year-old man a systolic blood pressure of 150 mmHg is common ('statistically normal') and asymptomatic ('clinically normal'), but his risk of a fatal heart attack is twice that of his contemporary with low blood pressure. Prognostically such values are abnormal.

4. *Operational*. However arbitrary, a decision must be taken that at some agreed level action is better than inaction. This operational definition of a case will take into account the clinical and prognostic definitions, but it may well differ from either: a person without symptoms may yet benefit from treatment, or another may have an increased risk that cannot be corrected. In screening, therefore, a case is defined as that level of disease above which action will improve either symptoms or prognosis, at an acceptable cost.

Quality control

Many doctors are unaware of the alarming results produced by quality control studies of bedside examination techniques. Table 3.1 shows results from a study in which three doctors were required independently to record opinions on the presence or absence of ankle pulses in a series of 96 patients. There was agreement in about three-quarters of cases. Perhaps the frequent lack of interest in such demonstrations of observer variation in clinical practice derives partly from a doctor's feeling that he is familiar with the dependability of his own physical findings, and his decisions are based on these rather than on the findings of his colleagues. For example, he may not be very concerned about the standardized grading of systolic murmurs because he knows the intensity which he personally regards as suspicious.

The laboratory services, especially in clinical chemistry, are more advanced in providing quality control checks. Standardization here is essential because a variety of technicians transmit results to a variety of users: if an outpatient on replacement therapy for hypothyroidism attends for periodic serum thyroid stimulating hormone estimations, it is essential that the values do not change simply because the laboratory engages a new technician. In the same way standardization and quality control are essential in epidemiological surveys. Because of their size these usually need to employ a number of observers in data collection, and

Table 3.1   Observer variation on the presence or absence of ankle pulses*

Pulse	Agreement on absence	Disagreement	Agreement on presence	Overall agreement
Posterior tibial	26	40	126	79%
Dorsalis pedis	28	59	105	69%

* Meade T W et al 1968 British Heart Journal 30: 661

furthermore a main objective is to compare results of different studies. In an investigation of respiratory function the rate of decline in forced expiratory volume over a period of years was shown to be much more rapid in cigarette smokers than in non-smokers. Such a conclusion was possible only because spirometric technique was rigorously standardized and observers were trained and regularly tested throughout the years of the study.

Figure 3.2 illustrates the frightening situation that can emerge if such precautions are not taken, even if the observers possess the highest professional skill and experience. Fourteen leading American cardiologists were each asked to assess the same 38 sets of pre- and post-exercise ECG tracings, and to record each time whether or not they saw evidence of ischaemia. Opinions ranged from that of the sanguine Dr N, who thought that only 5% were abnormal, to that of gloomy Dr F, who saw evidence of ischaemia in no less than 58%. One can imagine the confusion that would result if Dr N and Dr F were to conduct surveys on the frequency of heart disease in two different populations.

It is for this sort of reason that in epidemiology one needs to emphasize rigorous quality control of the main methods of measurement. This evaluation of methods implies two kinds of assessment, *repeatability* and *validity*, each of which has various components that it is important to distinguish.

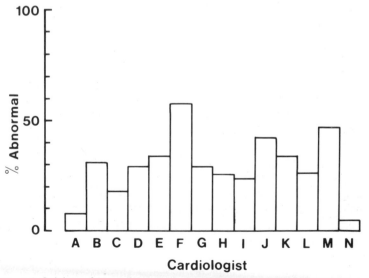

Fig. 3.2 Opinions of 14 cardiologists on the abnormality of post-exercise ECGs

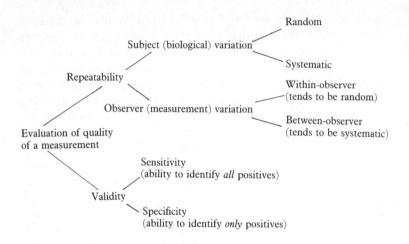

Repeatability

Repeatability is the level of agreement between replicate measurements, and it represents the degree of stability of both the subject and the observer (or the measurement technique). Cervical smears taken from the same woman on consecutive days may contain abnormal cells on one day but not on the other: this is *subject (biological) variation*. If the same smear is re-examined after an interval by the same technician, the two reports may differ: this is *within-observer variation*; it tends to be random or unpredictable. The likelihood of disagreement between two reports on the same specimen is greater if two different technicians report independently, since in addition to the inherent instability of each individual there is now the added factor of *between-observer variation*, due to systematic differences between them (see Fig. 3.2).

Random variation, whether originating in the subject or the observer, leads to misclassification of individuals, reducing the confidence that can be placed in each particular diagnostic assessment or report. Random variation is therefore important in clinical practice, where the individual is the unit of concern, but it matters less in epidemiology, where the unit of concern is generally the whole group or community. By definition random errors on average cancel out, and so they do not bias an estimate of the amount of disease in the group as a whole, provided that the group is reasonably large. Here lies a great strength of epidemiology: when statements are being made about the findings in a large group of people, random errors in individual measurements tend to cancel out, and a level of uncertainty in individual measurements is acceptable which in a clinical situation would be hazardous. This permits the use of simple methods of examination, so necessary in large studies in the general population. Coronary angiography may be the most accurate way of diagnosing coronary artery disease, but fortunately for the epidemiologist the frequency of the disease in different groups can reasonably be compared on the basis of a short self-administered chest pain questionnaire and an ordinary ECG.

There are, however, ways in which random measurement error arouses concern, and every survey should include some study of its magnitude. Poor repeatability may identify an inherently bad method or bad observer, pointing the need for improvement in either. It also introduces 'background noise' which, even though not biasing estimates of frequency, still tends to conceal or diminish associations. For instance, because of the large random errors in sphygmomanometry, the extent of familial aggregation in blood pressure was at first much underestimated: it blurred the true resemblance between relatives.

Fortunately the effects of random error can usually be much reduced by the simple expedients of making replicate measurements on each subject or enlarging the size of the study sample. The same cannot be said of *systematic measurement variation*. Of relatively less importance in clinical practice, its effects in epidemiology are drastic and largely irremediable. The dangerous bias which Dr N and Dr F (see Fig. 3.2) would bring to an epidemiological comparison would be in no way lessened by increasing the sample size, since error would be built into the study. Faced with any report of an apparent difference in the amount of disease in two groups, it is advisable first to look closely for evidence that the difference lies in the investigators rather than the populations.

Validity

Validity is the extent to which a technique measures what it purports to measure. What is its relation to repeatability? In a court of law if two witnesses disagree it can be concluded that at least one is false: poor repeatability necessarily implies poor validity. But if both witnesses agree it does not follow that they are truthful: they may be a pair of liars who have agreed on a false story. Hence a method that is repeatable is not necessarily valid.

Assessment of validity requires an independent standard of reference that can be accepted as trustworthy. Sometimes this is straightforward; for example, the validity of glycosuria as a measure of diabetes can be tested by comparing it with the glucose tolerance test. But sometimes it is more difficult: the validity of X-ray mammography in the diagnosis of breast cancer can be only partially assessed by comparing its verdicts with the results of biopsy. Biopsy detects only false positive errors, because biopsy of apparently normal women is impossible. To measure the validity of a chest pain questionnaire in the assessment of angina is harder still, for a positive result cannot be proved false even if coronary angiography was found to be normal. Validity is an important concept, especially in screening surveys, but its measurement can be difficult.

A valid measure of disease should have two characteristics: it should be both *sensitive* and *specific*. Sensitivity refers to its ability to detect a high proportion of the true cases, that is, to yield few false negative results. Specificity is the reverse: a specific test is one that correctly identifies the true negatives, and hence yields few false positive verdicts. Table 3.2 gives an example based on the performance of two alternative screening methods for breast cancer, namely mammography with or without clinical examination by a doctor. The tests were applied to 1500 women, of whom 16 proved to have breast cancer then or within the following 6 months. Mammography alone detected 9 of those 16 cases: this is the *sensitivity*, i.e. *the proportion of true positives correctly identified.* It was negative in 96% of the true negatives, and this figure is the *specificity*, i.e. *the proportion of true negatives correctly identified.* The same information could also be expressed as the 'false positive rate' (100 – specificity = 4%). Of the 69 with positive mammograms, only 9 proved to have cancer: this is the predictive value of a positive test, i.e. *the proportion of test positives that are true.*

These measures of validity indicate how a test will perform in practice, and they can also be used to compare alternative tests. In the example given, the combination of a clinical examination with mammography improved the sensitivity but at a price of many more false positives and a low predictive value.

The predictive significance of a positive test result can vary greatly according to circumstances. This arises because of the large overlap that commonly occurs between the distributions of 'true positives' and 'true negatives'. Consider for example the

Table 3.2 Performance of screening tests for breast cancer

	Cancer present	Cancer absent	Total
Mammography			
Positive	9	60	69
Negative	7	1424	1431
Total	16	1484	1500
Mammography + clinical examination			
Positive	13	150	163
Negative	3	1334	1337
Total	16	1484	1500

Proportion of true cases correctly identified (sensitivity)
  = 9/16 = 56% (mammography)
    13/16 = 81% (both together)
Proportion of true normals correctly identified (specificity)
  = 1424/1484 = 96% (mammography)
    1334/1484 = 90% (both together)
Proportion of test positives that are true (predictive value)
  = 9/69 = 13% (mammography)
    13/163 = 8% (both together)

electrocardiographic finding of a Q-wave of moderate size (e.g. 0.03″ in duration in lead aVL). Among patients with myocardial infarction this is common, but exceptionally it may also occur in people with normal hearts. The familiar clinical interpretation of its significance comes from experience of situations where most hearts are diseased; and even if, say, 1 per cent of normal hearts are associated with a Q-wave of this size, these 'false positives' will be greatly outnumbered in clinical practice by 'true positives'. The situation is quite different in a population survey or in routine screening. Here the proportion of 'true positives' could easily be as low as the proportion of 'false positives'. Thus in the hospital situation the finding of a moderate sized Q-wave is of high diagnostic significance; in the community exactly the same finding is as likely as not to be physiological. Put in general terms, the predictive (diagnostic) significance of a clinical finding depends on the frequency of disease in the situation where it is recorded (see also p. 131).

Often a test can be modified in order to improve its sensitivity, for example by combining mammography with clinical examination of the breast. Unfortunately, as false negatives diminish false positives tend to increase; and tests are often made more sensitive only at the cost of making them less specific. The problems of balancing sensitivity and specificity in screening tests are discussed in Chapter 8.

Types of survey

The sources of information on the medical problems of a community form a hierarchy in which there is a progressive and often steep increase in complexity and costs. At the base of the hierarchy are routine statistics, which have been discussed already; above them are special *ad hoc* surveys, ranging from simple descriptive surveys based on groups of cases, to cross-sectional population surveys, and finally longitudinal population surveys and trials.

In themselves health statistics are useless and often uninteresting. One of their functions lies in providing an informed and rational basis for the improvement of health care: decisions on the best use of medical resources should be related to know-ledge of the community's health needs and of the benefits derived from different services. It is a function of epidemiology to supply this information, either from routine statistics or from special surveys. The importance of the particular decision at issue should decide how far any investigation needs to proceed, but the principle is to start with the most readily available data and then to proceed only as far as one must with special surveys. Valuable though it would be to have nationwide data on the frequency of all major diseases, this is unfortunately out of the question. Larger and more complex studies must be reserved for problems that merit high priority. Unfortunately this means that less critical decisions must often be based on evidence that is manifestly not ideal. For this reason it is important to be aware of the limitations as well as the scope of each kind of survey.

Simple descriptive surveys

The basic epidemiological description of a disease is derived from relating the characteristics of a group of cases, such as age, sex and occupation, to those of the population to which they belong. In countries where accurate censuses are carried out the necessary population data can be readily obtained, and the practical problem is one of defining the *related population*. A related population comprises all and only those individuals who are notionally at risk of contributing to the case series. Related populations may be defined by geographical location, by time-span (e.g. all births occurring during one year), or by the characteristics of people (e.g. age and sex). Where description of the disease requires population data other than that recorded in censuses, it will be necessary to make direct observations on a control sample of the population. This is one form of the case-control method. This method is used for aetiological as well as descriptive studies (the distinction between the two is not clear-cut), and the procedure for selecting controls is described in detail in Chapter 5.

The starting point in identifying cases is likely to be some sort of diagnostic register, which may or may not be complete. Since not all patients with the condition will be receiving medical care, there is selection on the ground of severity. In specialist hospitals, and hospitals in large cities, the situation may be further complicated: a particular kind of case may be preferentially referred, or patients coming from a distance may be drawn from higher socio-economic classes rather than lower. The conditions for epidemiological studies are often better in general practice, or where one hospital or group of hospitals serves the whole of a defined community.

Cross-sectional population surveys

These studies depend on a single examination of a cross-section of a population, in contrast with *longitudinal studies* which trace changes in a population over a period of time. The difference is that between a photograph and a ciné-film. Three kinds of aim may be distinguished: (1) *description* of the burden of a disease on the community, and its distribution; (2) *study of causes of disease* (see Ch. 5); and (3) *screening* for hitherto undiagnosed cases (see Ch. 8).

The essential difference between a simple descriptive study and a cross-sectional population survey is that in the latter the study group is a sample of a complete population; sick and healthy alike are caught in the survey net and are not distinguished until the results are examined. This at once solves some of the problems that beset studies in which the starting point is a case series, assembled from hospital or clinic records. In a population study the cases truly represent the disease in the whole community. Any contrasts between the cases and the healthy subjects cannot be the result of biased selection, neither are they likely to result from biased assessments, since at the time of examination the diagnosis is usually unknown and all subjects receive the same scrutiny.

The measure of disease frequency that cross-sectional studies yield is *prevalence*, the proportion of persons affected at the particular time when the community 'photograph' was taken. (The terms cross-sectional survey and prevalence survey are often used interchangeably.) This is appropriate as a measure of the community burden from a relatively stable chronic condition, such as chronic bronchitis or schizophrenia. But the probability of detecting a case of disease is related to the mean duration of the disease, and therefore the cross-sectional method is generally inappropriate to the study of acute conditions (infectious diseases, for example, or acute episodes of chronic diseases). Population surveys involving personal examination are also inappropriate to the study of uncommon disorders such as multiple sclerosis. For these diseases prevalence surveys depend on intensive case-finding within a defined population, using all possible sources of information, including hospital and general practice records and the registers of welfare and voluntary organizations. Observations on the cases are then related to data on the related population, derived either from censuses or from direct observations on samples.

The main stages in the design and conduct of a cross-sectional (prevalence) survey may be summarized as follows:

1. *A precise aim needs to be specified*, preferably one that is demonstrably relevant to some practical decision on disease control or management. Vague aims produce vague studies. Suppose, for instance, that the objective was to determine the prevalence of untreated hypertension in a district, as a prelude to planning a screening service. It would first be necessary to specify the exact definition of 'hypertension' for this purpose (related to the level that is thought to require treatment), and also the accuracy with which its prevalence needed to be known (since this determines the required size of the study sample). The costs in time, money and other resources should be estimated in advance, since it is wasteful to start a study unless it is reasonably sure to achieve its aim.

2. *Definition of the study population* is of central importance. The purpose of epidemiological studies is to measure the disease in a *population*. In epidemiology this means an entire group of persons identified by some defined natural characteristics which they have in common, such as area or type of residence, occupation, age and sex, etc. The epidemiologist uses the term population in a wider sense than the demographer, to whom it implies people living in a particular area. Both might speak of 'the population of England

and Wales', but the epidemiologist might also speak of studying 'a population of smokers' or 'a population of residents in old people's homes'.

For certain routine statistics, for example mortality, complete national coverage is possible; but in surveys involving personal examination information can usually be obtained only from a sample of the population, and from this small experience general inferences are drawn about the population as a whole. This is justifiable only if sampling has followed strict statistical principles, and even then care must be taken in extending generalization beyond the particular 'population' from which the sample is drawn. This is especially true of studies based on occupations, where factors related to health may influence both the choice of job and the probability of remaining within it.

3. *Sample size* must be considered early in the planning of any survey. Prevalence rates in the general community often prove to be unexpectedly low, even for the commoner diseases. It is frustrating to complete a study and then find that it identified only two or three cases of the condition. To avoid this error investigators must first decide not only what they want to measure, but how accurately they want to measure it. Suppose, for example, that one wishes to study the proportion of adults who regularly take analgesics. First one needs some approximate idea of the order of frequency to expect — available data suggest a figure of about 30%. Next a decision must be taken on the required accuracy of the prevalence estimate. The sample may chance to be unrepresentative, the size of this uncertainty being measured here by the *standard error of the prevalence rate:*

$$\text{s.e.} = \sqrt{\frac{p(100 - p)}{n}}$$

where p = per cent of affected persons
       n = number in sample

If one were to decide that an acceptable standard error (s.e.) would be 2.5%, this would imply that in 95% of samples of this size the actual result would be within about 5% ($\pm$ 2 s.e.) of the population value. With the prevalence estimate cited (30%) and the specified level of precision (s.e. 2.5%) it can readily be calculated from the formula that the required sample size is around 300.

It will be noted that the sampling error depends on the

prevalence of the condition, so that to obtain a given precision it is necessary to study larger samples for uncommon conditions (such as rheumatoid arthritis) than for common ones (such as migraine). It can also be seen that sampling error is proportional to the square root of sample size, so that doubling the sample size would increase precision only by a factor of 1.4. Small studies tend to lack *power* (that is, the ability to identify the true state of affairs); this can lead to falsely negative conclusions from comparisons or trials.

Surveys of continuously distributed variables, such as blood pressure or biochemical values, do not generally need to be so large as studies of the prevalence of 'disease', since every examined individual contributes a value to the total pool of information. For these variables the measure of sampling variation (the *standard error of the mean*) is given by:

$$\text{s.e.m.} = \sqrt{\frac{s^2}{n}}$$

where s = between-subject standard deviation (a measure of the variation between different people based on the scatter of individual measurements)
n = number of subjects

Again, the investigator must decide, in terms of the s.e.m., how accurately the mean value of the study variable needs to be assessed and, using results from previous studies, the approximate value for the between-subject standard deviation: the equation can then be solved for n. For blood pressure, 95% of samples of 50 subjects will have a mean that is about within 5 mmHg of the actual population mean.

It is hoped that these guidelines will be sufficient for sample size determination in a simple survey of the kind that a clinical doctor can undertake, for example a general practitioner studying the prevalence of cigarette smoking in different age and sex groups of patients, or a chemical pathologist establishing normal values in healthy subjects. For more ambitious studies it is well to seek professional statistical advice.

4. *Recruitment of sample.* Although use of *volunteers* is convenient it is unwise to base generalizations on them. People who volunteer for medical studies tend to be either hypochondriacs or aggressively healthy. If a chemical pathologist wishes to establish the normal range of serum thyroxine as measured by a new method, it is easier to study members of the laboratory staff than to leave the hospital in search of a more representative group.

Even if the investigator perseveres and gets as far as the local factory, it is easier to call for volunteers than to obtain a random sample. In one study, designed to establish the prevalence of antibodies in rheumatoid disease, the investigator stood on the hospital steps and invited passers-by to step inside. It would be unrealistic to assert that every statement about normal ranges or prevalence rates must be based on random population samples: life is too short. But anyone who takes a short cut should be aware of the risks involved, for volunteer samples have often proved to be seriously biased.

The principle of random sampling is that every person or other sampling unit (e.g. household or school) in the parent population must have a predetermined chance, usually an equal chance, of selection. The initial procedure is a complete enumeration of the whole population from which the sample is to be drawn, since only in this way can each individual (or unit) have a chance of selection. In a general practice equipped with an accurate and up-to-date age/sex register this is easy. In the case of a survey of, for instance, untreated hypertension in a hospital district, one would probably turn to the electoral register, although care would be needed to ensure that the hospital and electoral districts were coterminous, and that the register was up to date. Surveys based on occupational groups can use the factory payroll, and surveys of children can be based on school registers. Sometimes none of these solutions is appropriate (particularly, of course, in non-industrialized countries) and then a special census may be necessary.

When the population has been enumerated each individual is assigned a number, and a sample of the required size is then selected by use of a table of random numbers. This constitutes a *simple random sample*. *Systematic sampling*, for example by taking every *n*th person on a list, may be less troublesome, but a need for caution is emphasized by statisticians. For example, to select every *n*th person on an electoral register would lead to under-representation of members of the same family, since they will be grouped together on the list.

Enumeration of a population does not always have to be based on a listing. For instance, in order to obtain a representative sample of schoolchildren in a large city it would be more convenient first to draw a random sample of schools and then within each selected school to draw a sample of children, a process known as *multi-stage sampling*.

Another refinement is to draw a *stratified sample*. Suppose that a large office population is to be used to assess age and sex differences in the prevalence of hyperlipidaemias. In a simple random sample a quarter of the subjects might be young women; there would be a further large group of young men, a moderate number of elderly men and very few elderly women. In order to achieve a more even distribution of these various categories in the sample to be studied it would be better to divide the company's nominal roll into 'strata' according to sex and decade of age. Equal-sized random samples would then be drawn from within each stratum.

It will be clear that the subject of sampling is not an easy one. Correct procedure is vital to the success of any survey, and some professional advice will be helpful if anything ambitious is to be attempted.

Labour expended on drawing an ideal sample is wasted unless subsequently there is a high *response rate*. Participation is always voluntary, but it nevertheless depends largely on the amount of public relations groundwork and on the investigator's persistence: in most situations a poor response rate reflects more the inertia of the investigator than the stubbornness of the population.

What response rate is acceptable? For an uncommon condition a response rate of 85% might be unacceptable, because a handful of cases in the unexamined 15% might greatly alter the findings; on the other hand, in a survey of drinking habits this response might be considered good.

In addition to prevalence, the acceptable level of response depends on the amount of bias. Non-respondents, and late respondents, tend to differ from those who come at first invitation. Those who did not reply to the first British doctors' smoking study subsequently had a mortality rate 40% higher than those who returned their questionnaires. It is helpful to have some measure of the amount of such bias. Two approaches are possible. Firstly, a small random sample is drawn from the non-respondents, and particularly vigorous efforts are then made to encourage their participation, including home visits; the findings will indicate the extent of bias among non-respondents as a whole. Secondly, some information must be available for all persons listed in the study population; from this it will be possible to contrast respondents and non-respondents with respect to basic characteristics such as age, sex and residence.

5. *Examination methods*, and the importance of their evaluation

and standardization, have been discussed already. The ordinary methods of clinical history-taking and physical examination are open to observer variation, and should never be used in surveys. The history should be obtained by a standard questionnaire, based where possible on simple 'closed-ended' questions, for example 'Do you usually bring up phlegm from your chest first thing in the morning in winter?' rather than 'When do you bring up phlegm?' Questions that seem clear and unambiguous to the doctor often seem otherwise to the respondent, and a new questionnaire should always be pretested on a small scale before its use in the main study. Similarly the interviewers or examiners will need preliminary training and experience. With many questionnaires it is possible to avoid the problem of observer variation by the device of self-administration.

6. *Records.* Anyone who has tried to use ordinary clinical records for research problems will know the difficulties and frustrations of data retrieval. The problem is still greater in epidemiological surveys, because the number of subjects is larger. The design of the record form is crucial, and it must be laid out with a clear idea of exactly how the information is later to be extracted and analysed.

The aims of the design are to help standardization, speed, and accuracy in recording under field conditions, and coding and retrieval of results afterwards. Writing takes time, and, where possible, non-numerical information should be ringed or ticked rather than written out. The layout should facilitate subsequent numerical coding and data extraction, with one answer box for each item of information. Copying takes time and may introduce errors; if the record can be precoded, results may go straight to the analysis. An orderly and uncluttered layout makes for fewer mistakes, in both the field and the analysis: results should be vertically aligned on the right of the page, well separated from questions and instructions.

The record starts with the subject's serial number in the study, followed by sufficient personal identification to permit any planned follow-up (address for postal contact, full name, date of birth, and — if available — NHS number for later tracing of morbidity through general practitioners, or mortality through the NHS Central Registry). If general practitioner or hospital follow-up is envisaged, the subject's consent should be recorded on the initial record.

Records should be pretested, both in the field on representative subjects and in the office for subsequent coding and data extraction. It is impossible to foresee all the practical snags. In large studies the record design should be discussed with the statistician who will later be concerned in the analysis.

7. *Analysis* of the results of a cross-sectional survey can proceed in various ways. Prevalence rates can be estimated in the study population as a whole, either for comparison with the results of other studies or as a guide to the planning of medical services; rates in different sub-groups of the study population may be contrasted in order to identify high-risk groups or areas; aetiological hypotheses may be tested by comparing the characteristics of the sick and the healthy; or the results may be used simply to describe the range of 'normal variation' in the population. These various uses are discussed more fully in subsequent chapters.

The choice of the actual technique of data processing will depend on the size and complexity of the analysis. A study of 100 subjects, with 20 characteristics recorded on each, could be analysed by manual tabulation of results and use of a desk calculator. But in most surveys the data will be coded in a form suitable for computer analysis. If (as is usually the case) the data are likely to be used on more than one occasion, the first step will be to transfer them to magnetic disc or tape. Results can then be read off very rapidly from the disc or tape into the core of the computer for analysis. Library programs are widely available for the input and analysis of survey data.

Longitudinal population surveys

Repeated observations on a population, or a sample of it, over a period of time permit the measurement of: (1) the rate of occurrence of new cases (*incidence*); (2) natural history and outcome (Ch. 7); and (3) the association between initial characteristics and the risk of future disease. Major examples of longitudinal surveys include the National Survey of Health and Development, which has followed a large group of British children born in 1946 through to adulthood, analysing such problems as the association between maternal health and the subsequent physical and intellectual development of the child; and the Framingham Study, which has followed for more than 30 years the inhabitants of the small town of Framingham, Massachusetts, and has successfully identified risk factors for

Table 3.3   Body-weight and the risk of gallbladder disease*

Relative weight %	No. of new cases in next 10 years		Morbidity ratio (%)
	Observed	Expected	
<90	35	45.7	77
90–	45	57.6	78
100–	62	52.6	118
≥110	84	68.5	123

* Friedman G D et al 1966 Journal of Chronic Diseases 19: 273

coronary heart disease, stroke, gout and gallbladder disease. Table 3.3, presenting results from this study, shows the importance of relative body-weight as a risk factor for clinical gallbladder disease.

The follow-up may take one of several forms. The simplest is to use routinely collected morbidity or mortality information, such as sickness absence records in occupational groups. A number of British studies have used an excellent system based on the NHS Central Registry, which maintains an indexed file of the entire nation. The records of participants can be marked with a code for that particular study, and when any of them subsequently dies a copy of the death certificate is automatically sent to the investigator. School records have been used, for example in order to assess the long-term effects of obstetric complications on child growth and development.

Obviously the range and quality of follow-up information available from such routine sources is limited, and for more clinically detailed assessment some form of re-examination is necessary. This raises two special problems. The first arises because of the difficulty in an increasingly mobile population of maintaining contact with study subjects over a long period of time: losses to follow-up involve just the same risks of bias to the results as does non-response in cross-sectional studies. The second concerns the difficulty of maintaining stability of clinical and laboratory standards over a long period of time, particularly when staff may have changed.

Added to the methodological difficulties of follow-up, longitudinal surveys usually have an added problem of sample size. The surveys are often large, lengthy and complex, and so unfortunately their applications tend to be restricted to conditions with a relatively high incidence. Results may be useless unless the study yields a sufficient number of new cases. An investigator backed by large resources planned to set up a longitudinal study to identify precursors of sudden death from coronary heart disease. As a community problem sudden cardiac death is common, but to each individual subject the risk within any one year is extremely low, and the investigator was forced to conclude that a longitudinal study to identify the precursors of sudden death would have to be impossibly large.

Sometimes a low-cost follow-up system may permit a large study at reasonable expense. Such a system has been applied with conspicuous success in the study of occupational diseases, especially cancers. The method depends on the fact that many industries retain their old personnel records, and it is sometimes possible to identify the people working on particular processes as long as 20 or 30 years previously. By searching mortality and cancer registry records one may discover which of these people have since died of the disease in question. In this way mortality rates can be compared between people employed on the suspect process and their age-matched contemporaries employed on other processes in the same workplace. This approach has been fruitful, for example in regard to cancer in radiation workers and lung cancer in butchers. Its limitation is that it identifies a risk which operated years previously, and which may well have disappeared with subsequent changes in the industrial process. This brings to mind the disturbing thought that in 20 or more years from now epidemiologists will be identifying the delayed effects of today's environmental pollution.

4. Methods of description

Numbers and rates

The distinction between clinical and epidemiological surveys has already been made. Clinical surveys describe patients. Epidemiological surveys describe patients in relation to the population to which they belong. In a review of neurosurgical patients in Wessex it was found that among patients aged over 65 years with brain tumours there were 83 men and 105 women. When, however, the numbers of cases were related to the numbers of men and women over 65 in the Wessex population it was found that there were 7.3 cases per 10 000 men and only 5.9 cases per 10 000 women. This seeming paradox results from there being approximately twice as many women as men in this age group of the population. It is thus that epidemiology gives an altered perspective to purely clinical data.

In epidemiology the frequency of disease is expressed as rates in which the numbers of cases are the numerator and the related population the denominator. In general a rate may be defined as the number of people with a state related to a disease (e.g. a pathological lesion) or the number of events (e.g. deaths or admissions to hospital) in relation to the total population at risk. An exception to this definition is provided by *proportional rates* which express the number of cases of a disease in proportion to cases of all kinds treated or dying in the same hospital, clinic or area. These rates are used only when population data are unavailable. For example, in occupational studies it is sometimes difficult to define the occupational population that gave rise to cases of disease, and proportional analyses are therefore used.

In this chapter the use of rates is illustrated. A list of those in common use, together with their definitions, is given in the Appendix.

Prevalence and incidence rates

Figure 4.1 shows the varying frequency of multiple sclerosis recorded in surveys carried out in North America and Australia. In each survey a count was made of all persons known to have multiple sclerosis within a defined population at one point in time. The results of the surveys are expressed as *prevalence* rates, which are represented on the map by circles with diameters proportional to the prevalence in that area. As stated in Chapter 3, prevalence rates define the proportion of people in a population who are affected by a disease at one particular time.

The map shows that the prevalence rates are higher at greater latitudes; but before concluding that the frequency of multiple sclerosis does in fact have this remarkable relationship with distance from the equator it is necessary to examine the difficulties in interpretation of the data, which arise both from using

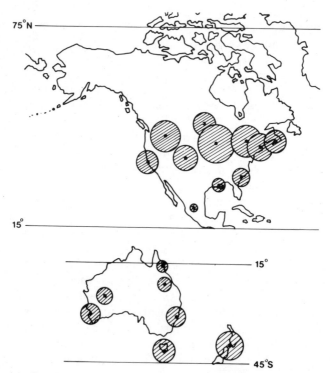

Fig. 4.1 Prevalence of multiple sclerosis in North America and Australia. (Source: Mathews W B (ed) 1985 McAlpine's multiple sclerosis. Churchill Livingstone, Edinburgh.)

prevalence as an index of disease frequency and from comparing studies of disease carried out in different areas.

The number of cases of a disease present in an area is compounded of the frequency with which new cases occur and are diagnosed (that is, the *incidence*) and the average duration before the disease is terminated either by recovery or death. This relationship between incidence and prevalence is illustrated diagrammatically in Figure 4.2. Prevalence rates may vary from one area to another solely because of variations in duration of the disease. It is likely that in non-industrialized societies, where infectious disease is widespread and the availability of medical care limited, multiple sclerosis will be more rapidly fatal. The prevalence of the disease will be reduced even if the incidence of new cases is the same.

Incidence rates express the rate of occurrence of new cases of a disease and may be defined as the frequency of some event related to a disease (e.g. onset of symptoms, hospital admission) related to the size of the population and a specified period of time. Most published incidence figures are annual incidences, but incidence may be measured over any period of time. Incidence rates have an advantage over prevalence rates in being uninfluenced by duration of the disease. During an epidemic influenza may have a high monthly incidence, but since the course of the disease is usually swift, the prevalence of cases on any one day will be considerably less than this monthly incidence. On the other hand for a chronic disease such as multiple sclerosis the annual incidence is much below the prevalence.

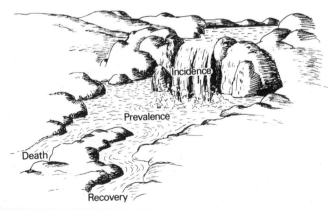

Fig. 4.2 Relationship between incidence and prevalence.

Although, ideally, Figure 4.1 would show incidence rates rather than prevalence, measurement of the incidence of multiple sclerosis raises formidable practical difficulties. Whereas prevalence can be measured by a cross-sectional study, completed within a few weeks, incidence requires a longitudinal study extending over months or years. Furthermore, since the prevalence of multiple sclerosis is greater than the annual incidence, use of incidence rates would require either surveys of larger populations or prolonged follow-up in order to obtain data of comparable accuracy. Other problems of measuring incidence include the frequent difficulty of dating the onset of symptoms and the variable delay between the onset of symptoms and diagnosis. For reasons of this kind the frequency of chronic diseases is often expressed as prevalence, and the use of incidence is restricted to acute conditions, such as many infectious diseases, or to acute episodes occurring in the course of chronic diseases.

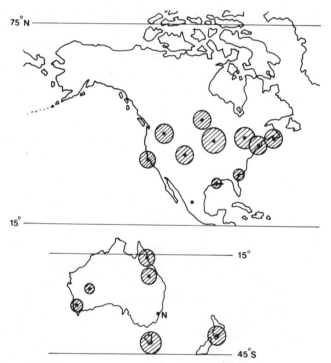

Fig. 4.3 Mortality from multiple sclerosis in North America and Australia. (Source: Mathews W B (ed) 1985) McAlpine's multiple sclerosis. Churchill Livingstone, Edinburgh.)

Figure 4.3 shows *mortality rates* from multiple sclerosis in selected areas of North America and Australia. As in Figure 4.1 the rates are represented by circles with diameters proportional to the mortality rate in that area. A mortality rate may be regarded as a form of incidence rate in which the event related to the disease is death. The mortality rates shown in the figure are annual rates but, as with incidence, mortality rates may be calculated for any period of time. Since few diseases are invariably fatal, mortality gives a distorted reflection of patterns of incidence: but since death is more likely to be reported than illness, mortality data are widely used.

It is now necessary to consider the difficulties of interpretation which arise when, as in Figures 4.1 and 4.3, maps of disease distribution are based on a number of separate surveys carried out by different observers using differing techniques.

Geographical distributions

When interpreting maps of disease distribution, on whatever kind of rate they are based, it is necessary to be aware of three influences that may distort a geographical distribution: (1) variations in levels of ascertainment; (2) variations in diagnostic criteria; and (3) variations in population structure.

The number of cases of a disease recorded by hospitals, general practitioners or in special surveys is partly determined by people's willingness and ability to seek medical attention. In countries with limited resources for medical care, variations in the level of ascertainment of disease from one area to another may be considerable, ascertainment often being better in the towns than in rural areas. In Britain, almost all cases of perforated appendix or fractured humerus will be ascertained, but the ascertainment of disorders such as depression or hypertension, which are not invariably disabling or fatal, may vary greatly between the Highlands of Scotland and the suburbs of London. Variations in ascertainment may also arise from differences in the quality of medical records. In international studies influences determining ascertainment always have to be considered before data from different countries are compared.

In epidemiological surveys the presence or absence of a disease is recorded using predetermined diagnostic criteria (see Ch. 3) and this standardization of diagnosis makes it possible to compare the results of one survey with another. However, in routine clinical work, diagnostic practice varies between one doctor and another. For example, some doctors may be more reluctant to diagnose an incurable disease such as multiple sclerosis in its early stages, or the frequency with which other diseases are initially misdiagnosed as multiple sclerosis may vary. Apparent geographical variations in prevalence or incidence can arise solely from such variations in diagnostic and recording procedures. Studies on death certification practices in different European countries have shown considerable international variation in the diagnostic descriptions recorded on the certificates of patients with similar disorders.

Throughout the world there are differences in population structure in terms of sex and age. The poorer, non-industrialized countries have a greater proportion of children in the population than do industrialized countries, where birth rates are lower and survival into adult life more usual. In Egypt, for example, 50% of the population is less than 20 years of age. Within Britain there are regional and local variations in the age and sex structure of the population and it is for this reason that age/sex standardized rates (see below) are widely used in geographical comparisons.

Both the prevalence and mortality maps for multiple sclerosis (Figs. 4.1 and 4.3) are based on data that are subject to error, but provided the magnitude of the errors is similar data from different areas may be comparable. It is reassuring that although the figures for mortality are smaller than those for prevalence both maps show the same higher frequency of the disease with increasing latitude. When data from Europe, Japan and other parts of the world are considered also it seems that this relationship with latitude is a general one. The apparent correlation between frequency of multiple sclerosis and latitude seen on the maps is supported by formal statistical analysis, and possible biological explanations of this interesting observation are considered further in the next chapter.

Age/sex standardization

Figure 4.4 shows mortality from gastric cancer among men in England and Wales. In the map the mortality in each area has been expressed as a Standardized Mortality Ratio (SMR) and the outstanding feature is the concentration of higher mortality in the north and west, especially in Wales. The SMR is an age/sex standardized rate and the need for standardized rates arises from the uneven distribution of disease between the sexes and at

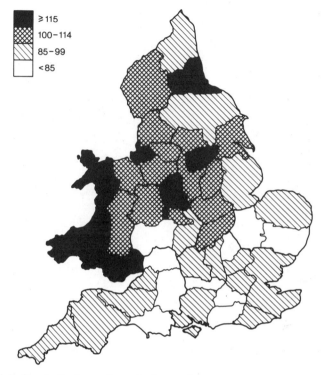

Fig. 4.4 Standardized mortality ratios for gastric cancer among men in England and Wales, (1979–85).

different ages, and from the variation in age/sex structure between one population and another.

Table 4.1 shows the number of male deaths occurring in Bournemouth and Southampton over a 5-year period, and the average annual death rates at different ages. The *crude death rate* (that is, the death rate at all ages combined) in Bournemouth (1694 per 100 000) is much higher than the rate in Southampton (1190 per 100 000). But inspection of the data reveals that Bournemouth has a greater proportion of old people in the population than Southampton, whereas the latter has higher death rates among old people. Clearly comparison of the total death rates requires a preliminary standardization for age. *Direct standardization* depends upon use of a population whose age structure is the standard. In this example the combined populations of Bournemouth and Southampton (166 221) are a suitable standard, although other populations could be used, for example those of one or other of

Table 4.1 Deaths in males in Bournemouth and Southampton over a 5-year period

a. Bournemouth

Age group	(1) No. deaths	(2) Population	(3) Average annual death rate per 100 000	(4) Annual no. deaths in combined population at Bournemouth rates	(5) Deaths in Bournemouth at combined population rates
Under 1	116	919	2524	71	22
1–44	204	34 616	118	116	38
45–64	1252	19 379	1292	566	264
65+	4076	11 760	6932	1447	869
Total	5648	66 674	1694	2200	1193

b. Southampton

Age group	(1) No. deaths	(2) Population	(3) Average annual death rate per 100 000	(4) Annual no. deaths in combined population at Southampton rates	(5) Deaths in Southampton at combined population rates
Under 1	223	1 897	2351	66	46
1–44	332	64 090	104	103	70
45–64	1728	24 440	1414	620	332
65+	3639	9 120	7980	1666	674
Total	5922	99 547	1190	2455	1122

the towns alone. To the standard population the age-specific death rates in the towns are applied (columns 4 in Table 4.1) giving an average annual total of 2200 deaths at Bournemouth rates and 2455 deaths at Southampton rates. These numbers of 'expected' deaths in the standard population give age-standardized average annual death rates of $2200 \times 100\,000/166\,221 = 1324$ per 100 000 (Bournemouth) and $2455 \times 100\,000/166\,221 = 1477$ per 100 000 (Southampton). The rate for Southampton is higher than that for Bournemouth, and the lower crude death rate in Southampton is seen to have been due to its smaller proportion of old people.

Indirect standardization depends upon use of standard age-specific rates. In this example the combined rates for Bournemouth and Southampton provide one possible standard. These rates are applied to the populations of the two towns (columns 5 in Table 4.1). A comparison is made between the average annual number of deaths that actually occurred in Bournemouth ($5648/5 = 1130$) and in Southampton ($5922/5 = 1184$) and the number 'expected' if the towns were exposed to standard rates (1193 and 1122 deaths respectively). This comparison gives standardized mortality ratios of $(100 \times 1130/1193) = 95\%$ for Bournemouth and $(100 \times 1184/1122) = 106\%$ for Southampton. Again a standardized comparison shows that mortality in Southampton is higher after allowance is made for the different age structure of the towns.

Distributions in time

Secular trends

Figure 4.5 shows the changing incidence of anencephalus reported from Dublin, Birmingham and Scotland over a 30-year period. Anencephalus is the second commonest cause of *stillbirth* (death after the 28th week of gestation) in England and Wales. In addition, since some anencephalics survive for a few hours after birth, it contributes to the total of *neonatal deaths* (deaths up to 28 days after birth). In the figure its incidence is expressed as the number of anencephalic births in relation to the number of *total births* (live births plus stillbirths). It may be seen that twice during 1936–65 the incidence of anencephalus in Dublin increased substantially and then declined. In Birmingham and Scotland there were also two rises in incidence which, although not as high as those in Dublin, occurred at approximately the same time. These interesting changes in incidence have evoked much

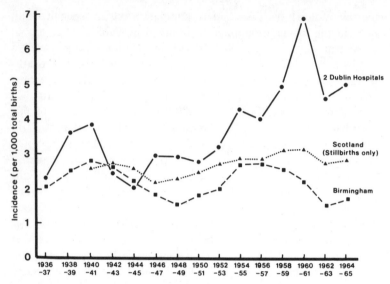

Fig. 4.5   Incidence of anencephalus reported from Dublin, Birmingham and Scotland, 1936–65. (Source: Leck I, Rogers S C 1967 British Journal of Preventive and Social Medicine 21: 177)

speculation on the aetiology of anencephalus. Changes in disease incidence of this kind, occurring over periods of many years, are referred to as *secular trends*.

As with geographical distributions, when interpreting secular trends three influences must be borne in mind: changes in levels of ascertainment, changes in diagnostic criteria, and changes in population structure. International comparisons suggest that the incidence of anencephalus in Irish hospitals is generally higher than in any other centres for which data are available, being between 4 and 7 per 1000 total births. The incidence reported from the two Dublin hospitals (Fig. 4.5) is somewhat lower than these figures, and the suggestion has been made that the apparent increase in incidence in Dublin to a peak in 1960–61 may have been the result of improvements in ascertainment and recording. It is impossible to disprove this suggestion, and the conclusion that there has been a true secular increase in anencephalus in Dublin rests on the magnitude of the increase and on detailed local knowledge of ascertainment and recording procedures in Dublin.

Fashions in diagnosis come and go. When death certification was introduced in England in 1838 deaths were attributed to 'privation' and 'old age'. Today deaths are attributed to 'strokes' and 'coronary heart disease', often on little evidence. With anencephalus, which is clinically obvious and invariably lethal, it is unlikely that changes in diagnostic criteria occur. But in demonstrating that the sharp increase in the recorded incidence of Crohn's disease in Britain during the 1960s reflected a true increase in disease frequency, it was essential to consider whether it could be accounted for by changing diagnostic practice, whereby certain cases hitherto classified as ulcerative colitis became diagnosed as Crohn's disease of the large bowel.

In Birmingham (Fig. 4.5) the second peak in incidence of anencephalus did not continue beyond 1957. It has been suggested that this may be attributed to the rise since that time in the proportion of children of non-European ethnic origin born in Birmingham, among whom anencephalus is relatively un-common. This suggestion illustrates the way in which changes in population structure may contribute to secular trends in incidence or prevalence.

Review of the data relating to the findings in Figure 4.5 has led to the conclusion that in Dublin, Scotland and Birmingham there have been fluctuations in the incidence of anencephalus since 1936 which at least in part are attributable to environmental influences common to all three localities.

Because of the scarcity of long-term morbidity data much of our knowledge of secular trends is based on trends of the underlying cause of death. These trends are influenced by changes in the rules for selecting one cause of death as the underlying one. In Britain during the Second World War deaths attributed to coronary heart disease fell in middle-aged people. This was attributed to the benefits of the war-time diet which was lower in fats and sugar and higher in cereals and vegetables, and was used as evidence to support dietary hypotheses for coronary heart disease. However, closer inspection of the data shows that in 1940 the rules for coding cause of death changed: where other diseases, particularly bronchitis, were recorded on the certificate they, rather than coronary heart disease, tended to be selected as the underlying cause of death. After allowing for this change in the rules there is little to suggest that time trends in coronary heart disease in Britain were much influenced by the war and the dietary changes that accompanied it.

Interpretation of secular trends is necessarily difficult. Whereas with geographical distributions the effect of variations in ascertainment, diagnosis and population structure are accessible

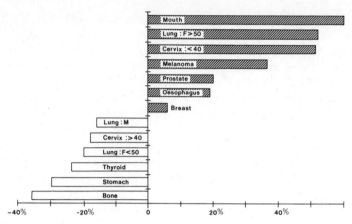

Fig. 4.6 Changing age-standardized mortality data from some common malignancies in England and Wales. The 1980–84 rates are expressed as a percentage of the 1970–74 rates.

to current enquiry, interpretation of secular changes depends upon observations made many years ago. Nevertheless the reality if not the true size of secular trends in disease frequency can sometimes be established with reasonable certainty. There is little doubt that the sharp increase in numbers of reported lung cancer deaths in England and Wales during this century resulted largely from a real increase in lung cancer incidence. Studies of the epidemiology of other cancers suggest that many of them are currently undergoing changes in incidence (Fig. 4.6).

Cyclic changes

Figure 4.7 shows the monthly variation in numbers of new cases of thyrotoxicosis diagnosed in selected areas of Britain. The numbers are above the average during each month from April to September. This represents a 6-monthly incidence of 13.8 per 100 000 population compared with 8.9 during the winter months, October to March. Figure 4.7 also shows the mean iodine content of milk. Iodine is contained in milk mainly because of its addition to cattle feed. Given that the median interval between onset of symptoms of thyrotoxicosis and diagnosis of the disorder was 12 weeks, the data are consistent with triggering of the disease by high winter milk iodine levels. They suggest that control of milk iodine levels in winter in northern countries may now be necessary.

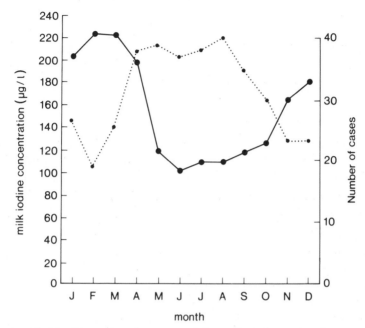

Fig. 4.7 Monthly number of new cases of thyrotoxicosis (● ----- ●) and average iodine content of milk (● —— ●) in selected areas of Britain.

The seasonal variation in incidence of thyrotoxicosis is an example of a *cyclic change* in disease frequency. Many diseases are observed to undergo regular cyclical changes. The onset of intussusception occurs more frequently during the day than at night. Sickness absence from work varies markedly with day of the week, with more people being absent on Monday than on other days: in contrast, sickness absence from school is most frequent on Fridays. The onset of wheezing due to byssinosis is characteristically on a Monday after a weekend away from exposure to cotton dust. The study of seasonal variation in incidence has always been important in infectious disease epidemiology, for the transmission of many viral, bacterial and parasitic diseases is seasonal. Other infectious diseases such as measles may occur in cycles of several years, since a lapse of years is necessary after an outbreak before sufficient non-immune children have been born to allow a further outbreak.

Many diseases whose aetiology is at present unknown have been found to undergo seasonal fluctuations in frequency and the interpretation of these observations is considered further in

Chapter 5. Description of secular, cyclic, or epidemic changes (discussed in Ch. 9) requires incidence rather than prevalence data. Usually incidence is related to time of onset of the disease (if there are reliable data on this) rather than to later events such as time of diagnosis or admission to hospital.

Characteristics of individuals

In describing the epidemiology of a disease certain personal variables and attributes are commonly used for giving a profile of the cases. (An *attribute* is a quality or characteristic of a person.)

Age

A clinical view of the age distribution of a disease is based on the numbers of cases in different age groups rather than on rates. Indeed in many descriptions of case series the age distribution of the cases is mistakenly called the age incidence, thereby confounding numbers of cases and rates. Figure 4.8 shows the age distribution of deaths from malignant disease of bone among elderly people in England and Wales. There is a peak in the number of deaths at age 70–74 years, with fewer deaths in younger and older age groups. Also shown are the same data expressed as death rates at each age. The death rates rise progressively with increasing age and there is no decline after the age of 70 years. Clearly the peak in numbers of deaths, which would be observed clinically, reflects the small numbers of very old people in the

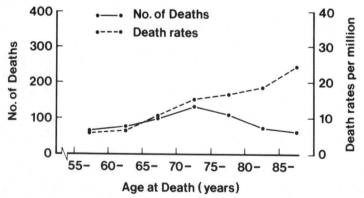

Fig. 4.8 Numbers of deaths and death rates from malignant bone tumours in England and Wales, 1982–85.

population, who therefore contribute only a few deaths to the total despite their higher death rates.

The apparent age distribution of a disease may be influenced by variations in ascertainment and diagnostic practice at different ages. Ascertainment of disease is often less complete among older people, and since prolonged and extensive investigation is sometimes contra-indicated in the elderly, their illnesses may be diagnosed with less precision than those of younger people.

When ages are to be grouped, the conventional groups are 0–4, 5–9, 10–14, 15–19 years, etc. It causes confusion to use different systems (6–10, 11–14, etc.), by making it hard to compare different case series. When ages are grouped in decades the groups should be 25–34, 35–44, etc., in order to minimize errors that result when inexactly known ages are rounded off to a multiple of 10.

Sex

The example of brain tumours among the elderly cited earlier (p. 49) points to the need to consider the sex as well as age distributions of disease in terms of rates. In Britain death rates from all causes are higher in men than women at each age, so that although at birth there are more males than females (about 105:100) among the elderly there are many more women. A disease of which there are more cases among elderly women than men may, in fact, have higher rates among males. Higher male death rates are particularly evident for coronary heart disease, chronic bronchitis, lung cancer and accidents. This is partly offset by female deaths from carcinoma of the breast.

Although overall mortality is higher among men, analysis of general practitioner consultations, sickness absence and hospital admissions suggests that morbidity is higher among women. This sex difference implies either that women have a higher incidence of non-fatal illness (diabetes and thyroid disease are examples of two common disorders known to be more frequent among women) or that men are less likely to seek medical treatment when they are unwell. Population studies of arthritis have shown that, for a given degree of radiological change, women are more likely than men to report symptoms.

The apparent sex distribution of a disease may be influenced by differential use of medical facilities, a common phenomenon in many countries where women do not share equal social rights with men, and by greater diagnostic difficulty in one or other sex, gonorrhoea, for example, being more difficult to diagnose in women. True variations in disease frequency between the sexes can be due to physiological or other intrinsic differences (as in cancer of the breast), or to behavioural differences. The male:female ratio of carcinoma of the oesophagus in Africa varies geographically from 12:1 to 1.5:1. It has been suggested that this correlates with differing cultural practices which determine whether or not women drink beer. Ingredients of beer are suspected as a cause of oesophageal cancer.

Socio-economic status

Living standards and lifestyle have profound effects on patterns of disease; indeed the improved standard of living resulting from the industrial revolution was probably the most important initiating factor in the decline in mortality in Britain which began in the nineteenth century and has continued until the present day.

In Britain the occupation of the head of the family has for 80 years been used by the Registrar General as an approximate measure of living standards. Occupations are graded into five classes according to their level of skill, financial rewards and the status they confer within the community.

Social class 1   Higher professional and administrative occupations
Social class 2   Lesser professional occupations and employers in industry and retail trades
Social class 3   Skilled occupations: N, non-manual; M, manual
Social class 4   Partly skilled occupations
Social class 5   Unskilled occupations

The classification is crude and gives only a rough index of the many factors that contribute to living standards, for example housing, education, income, child-rearing practices and attitudes towards health. It also has the practical disadvantage that there are many more people in social class 3 than in any of the other classes, approximately half the population falling into this class. Nevertheless it has proved useful in practice and Table 4.2, showing the rise in mortality from subarachnoid and cerebral haemorrhage and cerebral thrombosis from the higher to the lower social classes, is one example of the many important inequalities in frequency of disease and death among people with different living standards.

Table 4.2 Standardized mortality ratios for subarachnoid and cerebral haemorrhage and cerebral thrombosis (males aged 20–64, Great Britain, 1979–83) according to social class

	Social class					
	1	2	3N	3M	4	5
Subarachnoid haemorrhage	66	79	97	115	111	154
Cerebral haemorrhage	72	78	91	104	118	170
Cerebral thrombosis	56	62	89	106	122	193

Table 4.3 Standardized mortality ratios (males aged 15–64, England and Wales) according to social class for five time periods

Time period	Social class					England and Wales
	1	2	3	4	5	
1930–32	90	94	97	102	111	100
1949–53	86	92	101	104	118	100
1959–63	76	81	100	103	143	100
1970–72	77	81	104	114	137	100
1979–83	66	76	99	116	165	100

Nearly all major causes of death in men increase progressively in frequency from social class 1 to social class 5, although a few diseases such as multiple sclerosis are more frequent among socially favoured groups. Table 4.3 shows mortality by social class, expressed as standardized mortality ratios, for five time periods. Within social class 1 the ratio has fallen in recent years, whereas in social class 5 it has increased; as a result the social class gradient has become appreciably steeper.

Occupation

On page 15 a brief account was given of the routine statistics collected on occupational mortality which reveal marked differences between men in occupations such as mining and glass-blowing on the one hand, and those in seemingly less dangerous occupations such as teaching or herding sheep on the other hand.

Certain occupations are known to be attended by special risks such as the development of mercurialism, or of bladder carcinoma following exposure to naphthylamines. But in many instances the association between occupation and disease is less direct. Some occupations may select people who are liable to or have already developed diseases. For example men who are registered as disabled are often employed as timekeepers or lift attendants. The high incidence of cirrhosis among publicans may be partly related to the attraction of the job to men who are already alcoholics, and men with chronic bronchitis will avoid jobs making heavy physical demands. Conversely the development of disease may lead to exclusion from certain occupations. Airline pilots must retire if symptoms or signs of myocardial ischaemia are found on routine health examinations. Occupations may determine the occurrence of disease through the socio-economic status and way of life that go with them as well as through the environment at work. A survey in Derbyshire showed that the wives of men working in dusty jobs, such as mining and foundry-working, had a higher prevalence of cough than the wives of those working in dust-free occupations. This suggests that part at least of the high prevalence of respiratory disability among men in dusty occupations relates to their living conditions rather than to the hazards of their work.

A bias in occupational health studies arises from the preferential recruitment of healthy men and women, whose disease rates are therefore below the average — the so-called *healthy worker effect.*

When a chronic disease causes slowly progressive disability, whether physical or mental, a person may be rendered unemployable at their original level of skill, and may gradually sink down the socio-economic scale. This phenomenon is known as *social drift*, and it contributes to the concentration of chronic disease and disability among the unskilled occupations. It is illustrated in Table 4.4 which shows the undue proportion of schizophrenic patients who belong to social classes 4 and 5 despite their origins from families in all classes.

Table 4.4 Social class distribution of schizophrenic patients, and the ratio of observed to expected number in each class for (a) the patients and (b) their fathers (at the time of the patients' birth)*

Social class	% of patients in class	Observed/expected no. Patients	Their fathers
1 + 2	9	0.6	1.1
3	50	0.9	1.0
4	15	2.3	1.0
5	25	2.3	0.9

* Goldberg E M, Morrison S L 1963 British Journal of Psychiatry 109:785

Indicators

In some circumstances direct measures of morbidity or mortality are not available and it is expedient to use indicators. These may be defined as readily available data which reflect a variable but are not direct measures of it. For example, the complications of peptic ulceration — perforation, gastrointestinal bleeding and pyloric obstruction — are usually dramatic events which bring a patient to medical attention and about which data are readily available. Description of their epidemiology in Britain has revealed remarkable geographical variations. Admission rates for perforated duodenal ulcer, for example, were higher in the more northerly region, Trent, and in urban areas (Table 4.5). There is also a declining secular trend and a cyclic trend which varies from one part of the UK to another. By implication these findings apply to peptic ulceration as a whole; but the epidemiology of uncomplicated peptic ulcer is largely remote from investigation because many patients have a mild, uncomplicated, self-healing ulcer that does not lead them to seek medical advice.

In the context of health in general, infant mortality rates have been widely used as indicators of the general level of health of a population.

Table 4.5 Annual hospital admission rates per 100 000 for perforated duodenal ulcer in two regions in Britain

	Men		Women	
Region	Urban	Rural	Urban	Rural
Trent	22.8	16.9	6.3	5.6
Wessex	13.0	7.8	5.1	3.7

Prevention of disease

5. Aetiology

Research carried out on patients is largely concerned with the later stages in the natural history of disease. When illness develops, an agent of disease (such as a microorganism) or an environmental influence (such as atmospheric pollution) has already interacted with the person, and the doctor's task is to forestall the progression of the illness or to arrest its course once it is established. In contrast, epidemiological research into aetiology relates to the early stages in the natural history of disease, and by identification of pathogenic agents and environmental influences it seeks to prevent their interaction with human populations.

The identification of circulating immune complexes in certain forms of glomerulonephritis helps to explain how the glomeruli become damaged: this is *pathogenesis*, and is part of clinical research. But it does not reveal why a few people have this particular immunological abnormality while most do not: this is *aetiology*, which requires study of the general population as well as patients.

Epidemiological studies may be broadly divided into three groups, each of which contributes a different kind of information about aetiology. In *descriptive* studies the frequency of occurrence of disease in different communities or in different subgroups within a community is described. *Analytic* studies are designed to test hypotheses about the influences that determine that some populations, or certain individuals within a population, are affected by a disease while others are not. *Experimental* studies test such hypotheses by showing whether or not the frequency of a disease may be changed by altering exposure to a suspected cause.

Clearly only certain kinds of causative influence are accessible to observation by epidemiological methods, but it must be borne in mind that no disease is the result of one influence alone. The concern of epidemiology is not to unravel the many interactions that result in illness but to identify those determinants that are susceptible of manipulation, and thereby to prevent disease. Epidemiological evidence about causation is often circumstantial and incomplete, but it is a guide to action.

Descriptive studies

Observation that the frequency of a disease differs from one community to another, or at different times, naturally leads to an attempt to correlate changes in disease frequency with changes in the frequency of a suspected cause. There is a high incidence of anencephalus in Ireland; the incidence of melanoma in Britain is increasing; the incidence of carcinoma of the stomach is declining. Such observations compel speculation about aetiology. But only exceptionally is such speculation fruitful by itself; the immediate revelation from a map of Africa that childhood lymphoma and malaria are geographically associated was exceptional.

More often, descriptive studies provide information that can be used to test aetiological hypotheses generated by other research methods. For example, among substances identified as having long-term toxic effects, only a few were first disclosed by epidemiological studies. Tobacco and naphthylamine (causing bladder cancer) are the two best-known examples. More often descriptive and epidemiological studies have been used to substantiate suspicions arising from other sources. A number of toxic effects have been disclosed first by clinicians or pathologists, for example vaginal carcinoma in childhood resulting from maternal stilboestrol therapy, pleural mesothelioma from asbestos, leukaemia in leather workers from benzene, nasal cancer from wood dust: fewer have been discovered by analogy with experimental work in animals, for example angiosarcoma of the liver resulting from vinyl chloride.

Geographical distributions

In Chapter 4 the world distribution of multiple sclerosis was considered and the conclusion reached that the disease becomes more frequent with increasing latitude. In seeking to explain this distribution there are three general lines of enquiry. Firstly, does the distribution reflect some characteristic of the ethnic groups inhabiting different parts of the world? Secondly, does it reflect variations in the biological, physical or chemical environment? Thirdly, does it reflect differences in the residential environment?

Data on multiple sclerosis show that it is common among the Dutch but uncommon in Afrikaaners; it occurs in American Blacks but has not been recorded in Africans; and American Blacks show the same greater frequency in the northern states as white people. Such observations as these show that the distribution of multiple sclerosis is not related primarily to the distribution of an ethnic group. It does not occur with similar frequency in all parts of the world inhabited by any one ethnic group, and within an area the frequency of the disease is generally similar in the various ethnic groups inhabiting it.

It has therefore been concluded that environmental influences must be critically important in determining whether the disease is common or rare. These influences could be related to the climate, soil composition, the occurrence of microorganisms, in fact to any part of the biological, physical and chemical environment. Alternatively they may be related to the residential environment. The slums of cities are one example of an unfavourable environment that results from the interplay of patterns of occupation, social relationships, housing, diet and many other factors; the epidemiology of vitamin D deficiency in childhood illustrates how critically some disorders are influenced by the residential environment.

To date the world map of multiple sclerosis has not been directly fruitful of a hypothesis to explain the distribution. Even so it is important as data against which hypotheses may be tested. For example, it has been suggested that the disease is due to an infectious agent, probably a virus, which usually occurs in some animal species and rarely is transmitted to humans. But no animal could be suggested with a distribution similar to that of the disease, and the hypothesis was not pursued.

Further insight into the influences determining geographical distributions is sometimes given by studies of *migrant populations*. Migrants leaving an area are freed from exposure to harmful environmental influences local to the area, but take with them the genetic determinants of disease and, for a varying period, any predisposition related to their social customs. For one generation they will manifest latent disease with a pathogenesis already initiated. Moving into a new area they bring a different pattern of immunity and through differing customs in such factors as diet and housing may have a different exposure to harmful influences in the new environment.

Studies of multiple sclerosis in South Africa have shown that among immigrants from the UK age-standardized prevalence rates are about 40 per 100 000 (rates similar to those of UK residents), while among whites born in South Africa the rate is only about 7 per 100 000. This finding suggests that an initiating factor acts some years before the onset of symptoms, and accordingly people migrating from the UK (an area of high incidence) to South Africa (an area of low incidence) take some of their higher risk with them. Studies of migrants offer at least the theoretical opportunity of estimating the latent period between an initiating event and the onset of symptoms.

As mentioned in Chapter 1, observation of disease incidence in migrant groups has been the basis of a number of studies of coronary heart disease, cancer and other common diseases. The interpretation of these observations is liable to certain difficulties. Migrants may be unrepresentative of the population they leave. In the studies of multiple sclerosis in South Africa it was necessary to exclude the possibility that immigrants from the UK included a disproportionate number of people who already had the disease and who hoped to benefit from a better climate. Migration itself subjects people to unusual stresses. It has been found that among Norwegian immigrants into the USA there is a higher incidence of psychosis than in Norway. Although this may point to environmental influences in the USA that lead to psychotic illness, it may also be a result of selective emigration from Norway of less stable persons more liable to mental illness, or of the unusual stresses imposed on immigrants during their adjustment to a foreign culture.

Distributions in time

Secular variations in disease incidence may result from social and cultural changes, or from changes in the biological, physical, chemical or residential environment. Interpretation of secular variations requires inferences to be made about changes that occurred many years ago, and it is often difficult to document adequately a past correlation between disease incidence and exposure to some disease agent or environmental influence. For example, the social class pattern of coronary heart disease seems to have undergone a major change during the last 50 years, but it

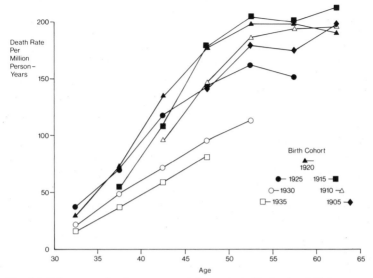

Fig. 5.1 Cohort mortality from cancer of the cervix in England and Wales

is impossible to relate this clearly to changes in diet, activity or other causative influences.

Whenever possible secular changes should be examined using age-specific rates. Figure 5.1 shows death rates from cancer of the cervix in successive generations, or cohorts, of women born in England and Wales. Generations have been defined by the midpoint in the range of years during which their members were born. Age-specific death rates change in successive generations. This is a so-called *cohort effect*. It suggests that successive generations have a changing exposure to some aetiological influence. Cancer of the cervix is associated with sexual activity and promiscuity, and the cohort effect can be interpreted in the light of this. For example, the generation that became young women during the Second World War was more sexually active, and had higher cervical cancer rates, than those which followed it. Cohort effects are distinguished from *period effects* caused by an influence, such as a change in treatment, which changes mortality in all age groups at the same time.

Many diseases with an aetiology at present unknown have been found to undergo seasonal fluctuations in frequency. While these observations may seem to provide a clue to the aetiology of the disease, their interpretation is necessarily difficult, for many potentially pathological influences vary with the season. Not only do the seasons influence the animal and plant environment, with changes in the availability of food and in the vectors and hosts of infectious agents, but there are seasonal changes in many aspects of human behaviour, such as occupation, diet and recreation. The effect of these changes on the body is seen in physiological variations: serum calcium levels, for example, tend to be lower in winter and early spring than at other times.

There is a higher incidence of congenital dislocation of the hip among infants born in the winter months. An explanation of this is that heavy bedclothes and consequent inhibition of infants' movement is a causative factor in the disease. This hypothesis is supported by the high incidence of congenital dislocation of the hip among Laps and American Indians who wrap their infants in swaddling clothes.

The winter excess of anencephalic births recorded in Scotland and other countries has led to a number of aetiological hypotheses, but none has yet been substantiated. It is of interest that in both Scotland and Birmingham the second peak in the secular trend shown in Figure 4.5 was due mainly to the increase in the anencephalus rate among summer births, which changed the seasonal pattern of incidence. Although the explanation of such observations may not be clear, they are nevertheless helpful in so far as hypotheses about causes may be untenable unless the suspected causes show corresponding cyclic variations.

Sometimes seasonal changes in disease frequency are explicable in terms of processes of little interest to the investigation of disease determinants. Data from several surveys have suggested that there are fewer births of mentally subnormal children in the winter months in Europe, and this has led to much speculation about seasonal influences that could damage the embryonic brain during the first months of pregnancy. However, it seems likely that this apparent fluctuation in the birth rate of subnormal children results from a raised mortality among children with congenital malformations born during the winter, such that more subnormal children born in winter die before their subnormality is recognized.

Disease incidence can vary with place or with time. Sometimes it varies simultaneously with both place and time. Movement of disease may occur in association with migration of people, or a disease may move through a static population leaving *clusters* of affected persons in its path. It is an easily recognized characteristic of many infectious diseases, from the common cold to smallpox, that cases occurring in any one place tend to occur at around the same time; this phenomenon has been termed *space-time clustering*. When several cases of uncommon diseases such as Hodgkin's disease or myelomatosis occur in a small area within a short time, they attract attention and may give the impression of an epidemic. However, apparent epidemics of this kind occur from time to time as a matter of chance, and it is through the use of cluster analysis that an attempt is made to determine whether the degree of clustering observed is such as is likely to occur by chance.

Great interest was aroused by the demonstration that, using such techniques, 96 cases of lymphoblastic leukaemia occurring in children in Northumberland and Durham showed evidence of clustering. Subsequent studies have provided conflicting results about clustering in leukaemia; but with another disease, Burkitt's lymphoma, clustering has been clearly demonstrated. One possible inference from this is that Burkitt's lymphoma is due to an infectious agent, and it is the possibility of revealing evidence of infectivity in diseases such as leukaemia and lymphoma that has stimulated the development of cluster analysis techniques. However, clustering may result from movements of aetiological influences other than microorganisms. Heroin addiction may show clustering as knowledge of the drug and its abuse spread in a community. The spread of new diagnostic interests and criteria, such as the diagnosis of Crohn's disease of the large bowel rather than ulcerative colitis, may also result in apparent clusters of cases. In this way a paper on milk allergy from Newcastle-upon-Tyne directly stimulated a local 'epidemic' of cot deaths ascribed to this cause: the total number of cot deaths did not vary, the only change being in diagnostic fashion.

Age distributions

The association of disease with personal characteristics such as age, sex and occupation has been considered in Chapter 4, but it is necessary to discuss further the interpretation of age distributions. The age at which a disease occurs reflects not only changes associated with ageing but also the differing experiences of different *age cohorts*. Within a population people of approximately the same age form an age cohort; such a group tends to share a similar environment from birth to death. Within the British population during the 1980s only people aged 60 years or more were alive when the pandemic of encephalitis lethargica reached its height in 1920, after which it declined almost to vanishing point over the next 15 years. Therefore, post-encephalitic parkinsonism today is an illness of older people, not because they are more susceptible to it but because they belong to age cohorts that were exposed to encephalitis.

Analytic studies

A broad distinction can be drawn between descriptive studies, presenting the occurrence and distribution of a disease, and analytic studies where the purpose is to test hypotheses about the causes of a disease. This distinction is not always a sharp one, for many studies provide both descriptive and analytic data, but it is useful in that analytic studies usually demand the use of controls, whereas descriptive studies do not.

Case-control and cohort studies

There are two kinds of epidemiological observations that are made on groups of individuals rather than populations, and provide evidence that a particular event (such as ingestion of thalidomide) or state (such as atmospheric pollution) may be a cause of a particular disease. As an example one may consider the evidence that implicated maternal rubella as a cause of congenital cataract.

1. *Comparison of people with the disease and normal people, showing that the suspected cause occurs more frequently among those with the disease than those without it.* An early Australian study showed that 68 out of 78 children with congenital cataract had a history of maternal rubella, whereas none of a group of normal children had this history.

2. *Comparison of people exposed to the suspected cause and those not exposed, showing that a greater proportion of people develop the disease among the exposed group than among the non-exposed.* In a study in Britain a group of women who suffered from rubella in pregnancy were followed up for two years after the birth of the child. One in six of the children whose mothers developed rubella during the first two months of pregnancy had a congenital deformity — a far higher incidence than that among children born after normal pregnancies.

Corresponding with these two types of observation there are

two methods used in analytic epidemiology. Case-control studies compare people with a disease and those without it. Cohort studies compare people exposed to the suspected cause and those not exposed.

The two types of study answer two different questions. To illustrate this, suppose that an investigation is required to determine whether delivery by forceps, and the accompanying trauma to the infant's head, can result in brain damage that is manifested as childhood epilepsy. A case-control study would involve comparing the obstetric histories of a group of epileptic children with those of a control group of non-epileptic children. The results can be expressed in a contingency table, where a, b, c, d represent the numbers of individuals in the four cells:

	Epilepsy	
	Present	Absent
Forceps delivery		
Present	a	b
Absent	c	d

If it were found that the proportion of epileptic children with a history of forceps delivery $a/(a + c)$ exceeded the proportion of control children $b/(b + d)$, this would suggest that forceps delivery is associated with and may be a cause of epilepsy. But there are many other determinants of epilepsy, so that among a group of epileptics only a small percentage of cases may be attributed to forceps delivery: this proportion is calculated from the difference between $a/(a + c)$ and $b/(b + d)$ which represents the relative contribution of forceps delivery to the total frequency of epilepsy. This is a guide to its importance as a community problem.

A cohort study of the same problem would compare a group of children delivered by forceps with a group of children delivered normally. The results can again be expressed in a '2 × 2' table. If it were found that the proportion of forceps-delivered children who developed epilepsy $a/(a + b)$ exceeded the proportion of normally delivered children $c/(c + d)$, this would suggest that forceps delivery is associated with and may be a cause of epilepsy. But forceps delivery does not invariably lead to epilepsy, which occurs in only a percentage of children delivered in this way. The difference between the incidence in the exposed $a/(a + b)$ and the incidence in the non-exposed $c/(c + d)$ represents the risk of epilepsy developing as a consequence of forceps delivery, and is known as the *excess* or *attributable risk*. This is a guide to the management of individual cases.

Both types of study may be used to show whether a disease and a suspected determinant are associated and therefore perhaps causally related. But analysis of this association by a case-control study will show the proportion of cases of the disease that may be caused by the determinant, whereas analysis by a cohort study will show the proportion of people in whom exposure to the determinant results in development of the disease.

The strength of a suspected cause can conveniently be expressed by its *relative risk* or *incidence ratio*:

$$\frac{\text{Incidence in exposed}}{\text{Incidence in non-exposed}}$$

In a cohort study this can be calculated directly, since the two incidence rates are known. In a case-control study the relative risk can be estimated only indirectly: under most circumstances this estimate will not differ greatly from that obtained in a cohort study.

Some writers use the terms *prospective* and *retrospective* study instead of cohort and case-control study. The underlying concept is that cohort studies are forward looking, in that they start with people exposed to the suspected cause, whereas case-control studies look backward, from people with the disease to suspected causes that have already acted. Unfortunately epidemiologists use prospective and retrospective both in this sense and in the more precise dictionary usage, whereby observations are said to be recorded prospectively or retrospectively according to whether they were planned in advance and collected at the time of the particular event (for example by interview of patients during admission to hospital), or whether they were recorded after the event occurred (for example from study of hospital case notes). The terms cohort and case-control avoid this possible confusion of meanings.

A further source of confusion is that the terms *longitudinal* study and *cohort* study are sometimes used interchangeably. In this text descriptive studies in which a population is observed over a prolonged period are termed longitudinal studies (p. 46). By contrast studies are termed cohort studies when they are designed to test a specific aetiological hypothesis and when the aetiological influences being investigated are the basis of cohort selection.

In the choice between case-control or cohort methods their relative feasibility is often the dominant consideration. Case-control studies may be carried out quickly and cheaply since groups of cases may be readily collected from hospitals and general practices. An association between laryngeal carcinoma and a history of exposure to asbestos was suggested by a study in which the case series was 100 consecutive men with laryngeal carcinoma attending one hospital, and the controls were 100 men with other diseases attending the same hospital. However, the annual incidence of laryngeal carcinoma is approximately 1 in 50 000; since many industrial workers are exposed to asbestos this low incidence suggests that if the disease occurs as a consequence of asbestos exposure it does so uncommonly. In these circumstances comparison of the incidence in a cohort exposed to asbestos and a non-exposed cohort may require many thousands of participants. Even if it were possible to collect a population of asbestos workers large enough to produce sufficient cases of laryngeal carcinoma for comparison, such a project would clearly be expensive and would be undertaken only by people with a full-time commitment to it.

If data on both the suspected cause and the occurrence of disease are available from routine data then large cohorts may be studied without prohibitive expense. In a study in Israel 11 000 children irradiated for ringworm and two control groups totalling 16 000 children were identified from treatment records of immigrants. The incidence of tumours of the head and neck over the ensuing 12 to 23 years was determined from a cancer registry file and from death certificates. Despite the large size of the cohort and the duration of follow-up such a study (which showed a higher risk of tumour in the irradiated group) could be carried out without massive resources. Likewise, if a disease has a high incidence and a short latent period, cohort studies may be both swift and inexpensive.

In addition to the feasibility of the two methods the kind of information they yield will also determine which is used. When clinicians noticed that many patients with chronic renal disease had a history of phenacetin ingestion there was evident need for cohort studies to determine the attributable risk. The findings of these studies suggested that renal failure is an uncommon sequel to high analgesic consumption, albeit phenacetin is incriminated to a degree meriting its withdrawal from use.

In summary the essential differences between case-control and cohort studies are as follows. Case-control studies depend upon comparison of people with a disease and those without it; they define the relative contribution of an aetiological influence to the total frequency of the disease; they can usually be carried out swiftly and inexpensively. Cohort studies depend on comparison of people exposed to a suspected cause of disease and those not exposed; they define the attributable risk of developing the disease following exposure to the cause; they tend to be time-consuming and costly. Generally case-control studies are used for exploratory investigation, and it is a particular strength of the method that a single study can simultaneously explore several causal hypotheses. Cohort studies are usually reserved for testing of precisely formulated hypotheses, since the suspected cause must form the basis for cohort selection and the expense and work required for the study can be justified only by detailed consideration of the likely outcome.

Execution of studies

The dominant practical consideration in most cohort studies is that they are prolonged. This is because in most chronic diseases the interval between exposure to a causal agent and mani-festation of the disease is long. Avoidance of a prolonged follow-up period depends on the good fortune of locating stored information on previous exposure that is relevant to the hypothesis being tested — as occurred in the study of irradiation and brain tumours already cited, and not infrequently occurs in industrial cohort studies, where factories are found to have employment records going back many years. For prolonged studies it is essential to select a cohort that is: (a) stable (not liable to substantial migrations) and therefore available for observation over the required period; (b) co-operative and likely to remain so throughout the study; and (c) easily accessible to the investigator so that the expense and labour of the study are minimized.

The size of the study cohort (that is, the cohort exposed to the suspected cause) will be determined by the estimated incidence in the unexposed population and by the minimum attributable risk that it is intended to detect. Detection of small differences in disease incidence between exposed and non-exposed cohorts will require either larger cohorts or more prolonged follow-up than detection of large differences. Statistical advice is an essential preliminary to the considerable investment of time and money entailed in a cohort study.

In a case-control study the two most immediate decisions are often the definition of a case (see p. 30) and the source of cases to be used. Incidence, i.e. newly diagnosed, cases are usually preferred to prevalence, i.e. existing, cases. Since for incidence cases the time of exposure to the suspected cause is generally more recent than for prevalence cases, the patients' recall of exposure will be better and so too will be the availability of any records of it. Occurrence of the disease may alter a patient's lifestyle, and the consequences of a disease may therefore be confused with its causes. For example, a study of diet in the aetiology of peptic ulcer would be difficult to interpret if prevalence cases were used because occurrence of an ulcer leads to various and unpredictable changes in dietary habits. Prevalence cases represent the survivors from all incidence cases, and factors influencing survival may be mistaken for causes of the disease.

Cases may be ascertained from clinic or hospital records or may be identified during a preliminary incidence or prevalence study.

Analytic studies utilize the same techniques of recruitment of participants, record design, examination methods and data handling as were described in Chapter 3. A crucial part of the methodology of analytic studies is the need to ensure that observations made on study cohorts or cases are directly comparable to those made on the controls, thereby avoiding bias (see p. 89).

Selection of controls

As has been mentioned already, analytic studies usually require control groups. The selection of controls is an exacting procedure, which requires careful planning.

At the outset it must be noted that the word control is being used in a particular sense. A biochemist seeking to determine the 'normal' range of values for a new blood test will require specimens from a group of 'controls'. Ideally specimens would be obtained from a random sample of the population, and a practical difficulty is to ensure that the actual group of people used as controls, for example patients or hospital staff, are not so unrepresentative of the population at large that measurements made on them will differ markedly from population values.

However, in aetiological studies the difficulty is that the control groups required are not random samples of the population, because some form of *matching* of study and control groups is almost always necessary.

Cohort studies. It is convenient to consider the choice of controls in cohort studies in relation to a specific example, such as an investigation of the association between oral contraceptives and deep vein thrombosis of the legs. The ideal method of investigating this association would be a trial, in which members of an 'experimental population' would be allocated at random, either to a group taking oral contraceptives or to a control group not taking them. But clearly such a trial is impracticable. The aim of a cohort study is analogous to a formal trial but has one essential difference: namely, individuals are not randomly allocated to the study cohort, taking contraceptives, but become members of it through the operation of cultural and social influences. In so far as these influences are also related to the development of thromboembolic disease they will affect the comparison between study and control cohorts.

To take a hypothetical example, if oral contraceptives are generally not used by social classes 4 and 5, and if these social classes also experience a lower incidence of deep vein thrombosis for dietary or some other reason, then a control group comprising a random sample of all social classes will have a lower incidence of deep vein thrombosis than the study cohort, independently of any association between the disease and contraceptives. In these circumstances social class is described as a *confounding variable* — a variable that is associated with the suspected cause and which, independently, determines disease risk. It therefore offers an alternative explanation to the study hypothesis. Although allowance for the influence of social class might be made by some form of standardization during the analysis, it would be more efficient if, at the outset of the study, the control cohort were selected to eliminate this influence.

The main criterion for selection of controls in cohort studies is therefore that, in so far as knowledge of the disease permits, the study and control cohorts should be equally susceptible to the disease. In the example being considered this requires that the two cohorts are matched in respect of variables such as age and parity which influence the frequency of deep vein thrombosis. Such matching will necessarily result in a control group that is an unrepresentative sample of all women in the general population in respect of age, parity and the other matched variables.

Having ensured that the control cohort has the required resemblance to the study cohort, it is also necessary to ensure that observations on the controls are made under the same conditions as those on the study cohort. Obviously it would be incorrect if the incidence of deep vein thrombosis in the study cohort were determined by periodic interrogations of the women, while that in the control cohort depended solely on inspection of hospital records.

The cohort method has been frequently used in the study of occupational disease. Sometimes one occupational group may be used as the control for another group in the same industry who are exposed to a suspected industrial hazard. Alternatively control data may come from varying levels or durations of exposure to a suspected cause within a single cohort, a technique used in studies of the relation between coal-miners' pneumoconiosis and exposure to different levels of dust among miners with different tasks. National statistics may be used as control data, especially for diseases with a high mortality, and knowledge of the hazards of bladder cancer in the chemical, rubber and cable industries has come partly from comparisons with suitably standardized national mortality rates. However, comparison of the health of occupational groups with national statistics must take account of associations between occupation and disease such as were mentioned in Chapter 4. Ill-health may cause retirement from many occupations, with the consequence that morbidity and mortality among those employed is better than the national average. On the other hand, some occupations select people who are liable to or have already developed diseases.

Case-control studies. Despite the apparent practical simplicity of the method the theory of case-control study design is complex and as yet imperfectly understood. A main difficulty lies in the selection of controls.

Suppose that an investigator wishes to compare the proportion of women with deep vein thrombosis who take oral contraceptives with the proportion in a control group. An initial response to the problem of defining appropriate controls may be to select them by random sampling from the same population as that to which the cases belong. If, for example, the cases are all patients within a group practice, then a random sample of all women of child-bearing age on the practice lists would be used. However, the results of such a case-control comparison would be difficult to interpret. If a greater proportion of the cases were found to be taking contraceptives there would be several possible explanations other than that the contraceptives are causally related to thrombosis. There may be confounding variables, such as socioeconomic influences, associated independently with the occurrence of thrombosis and the use of contraceptives.

It is because confounding variables are usual in associations between diseases and their causes that random sampling of populations to obtain controls does not permit critical examination of a suspected cause, unless the size of the control group is such as to permit the effects of confounding variables to be explored during the analysis. It is often more efficient to match cases and controls in respect of confounding variables at the outset of the study.

Detailed exposition of the principles of matching is beyond the compass of this book, and it must suffice here to state that there are three kinds of variable (or attribute) on which controls could be matched with cases. Firstly, there are variables that are associated with exposure to the suspected cause but not, independently, with development of the disease. Religious belief may determine the acceptability of oral contraceptives but is generally unlikely to have an independent association with deep vein thrombosis. Matching on such variables tends to conceal the association being investigated. In an extreme case perfect matching of influences that determine exposure to the suspected cause will result in the frequency of exposure in cases and controls becoming identical. This is over-matching.

Secondly, there are variables associated with the development of the disease but not with exposure to the suspected cause. The presence of varicose veins increases the frequency of venous thrombosis but probably does not often influence whether a woman takes oral contraceptives. Matching on such variables is generally without effect, altering neither the validity nor the statistical efficiency of the comparison.

Thirdly, there are the confounding variables, which are associated with both exposure to the suspected cause and, independently, with the development of the disease. Age and sex are obvious examples in relation to oral contraceptives and deep vein thrombosis; there must indeed be few causes or diseases that are not influenced by age and sex. In respect of such variables either cases and controls must be matched or allowance made for them during the analysis. When controls are matched to cases on, for example, sex and three categories of age, the six age/sex groups are referred to as *matching strata*.

Matching may be carried out either in groups, so that the overall distribution of confounding variables is the same among the cases and controls, or by individual, so that each case is matched to one or more individual controls.

Although the cases in case-control studies are not usually selected from a precisely defined population, it is useful to consider that they belong to a hypothetical one, comprising all individuals who, if they developed the disease, would be included as cases but are otherwise potential controls. The choice of controls is dictated by the need to have individuals without the disease who are representative (in respect of exposure to the suspected cause) of the population within the population matching strata selected, e.g. age/sex/social class groups.

In practice the number of potential controls is often limited and the constraints of rigorous matching criteria may lead to insufficient controls being available. Sometimes, if individual matching is restricted to the dominant confounding variables, it is possible to allow for other variables by group matching during the analysis. At other times the investigator may have to accept that the number of confounding variables is such that the case-control method is not feasible.

The *sources of controls* in case-control studies include patients, relatives, neighbours and the general population. The choice of a source is mainly determined by the need for cases and controls to have certain similarities and for observations on controls to be made under the same conditions as those on cases.

Since many case-control studies depend upon the investigation of hospital patients it is often convenient to select a control group from other patients in the same hospital. However, patients with some diseases may be unsuitable as controls because the diseases have a positive or negative association with the suspected cause, thus making the patients unrepresentative of the population in respect of exposure to the suspected cause. A study of the relationship between cigarette smoking and bladder cancer was rightly criticized because the controls were drawn from a respiratory clinic. This violates the principle that controls must be representative of the population within the particular matching strata being used, and is an example of selection bias (see p. 89). Because of the possibility of an unforeseen association between a disease and a suspected cause it is usual to choose control groups from patients with a variety of diseases.

The relatives of patients may form an appropriate and accessible group from which controls may be selected. Relatives not only have genetic similarity but tend to share a common environment.

In studies of influences determining intelligence relatives have often been used. The average IQ of a group of 1338 children whose mothers were anaemic during the pregnancy was found to be below average at 97.4. But since anaemia of pregnancy occurs more often in families where the general level of education and measured intelligence are low, it cannot be concluded that anaemia is causally related to the reduced mean intelligence. Resolution of this difficulty in interpretation required matching out of the confounding socio-economic variables related to anaemia (the suspected cause) and lowered intelligence (the disease). This was most readily achieved by use of a control group comprising brothers and sisters of the children. The mean IQ of children born after pregnancies complicated by anaemia was the same as that of their brothers and sisters born after uncomplicated pregnancies.

When confounding variables are geographically localized, for example variables related to quality of housing, then matching of cases and controls may be most readily accomplished by use of neighbours as controls. This method is often used in non-industrialized countries where the absence of listings of the population, such as electoral rolls and general practice registers, or of precise addresses make other methods of selecting individuals from the general population difficult.

When controls are drawn from the general population it is often necessary to use some form of sampling (see p. 41). Likewise when controls are drawn from groups of patients or relatives, the manner of selection should be defined and orderly, e.g. consecutive admissions or consultations, rather than based on convenience. The use of 'healthy volunteers' is likely to introduce bias and is rarely satisfactory.

Interpretation of data

In general the outcome of an analytic study is the conclusion that a disease and its suspected cause are or are not *associated*. The simplest method of presenting an association is by means of a '2 × 2' table, as shown in Table 5.1. Such tables are concise and easy to analyse statistically, but are appropriate only if the disease and suspected cause can be recorded as present or absent, i.e. if the data are *qualitative*, having no statement of magnitude. If the data are *quantitative*, being derived from measurements on a scale, such as haemoglobin concentration or levels of atmospheric pollution, then demonstration of an association will require

Table 5.1 History of therapy with conjugated oestrogens in patients with endometrial carcinoma and matched controls

	Patients		Controls	
	No.	%	No.	%
Oestrogen therapy	54	57	29	15
No oestrogen therapy	40	43	159	85
Total	94		188	

tabulation of grouped data or use of statistical indices such as the correlation coefficient (see p. 91).

Interpretation of data of the kind shown in Table 5.1 requires that three questions be answered. Firstly, could the apparent association be the result of some bias in the investigation? Secondly, is it likely that chance alone could produce the observed association? Thirdly, if the association is real, is it most reasonably explained on the basis of a cause-and-effect relationship?

Bias in analytic studies has two main forms. In the case-control study of endometrial carcinoma an obvious possible source of bias, which was taken into account during execution of the study, was that data on oestrogen therapy were obtained retrospectively from clinic records. Patients with endometrial cancer might have been exposed to a more probing and thorough enquiry about their history of oestrogen therapy than the controls, who were patients attending the clinic for a variety of other disorders. This is an example of what has been called *ascertainment bias*, which arises when information obtained from cases and controls is dissimilar in quality or source.

Selection bias arises when controls, or cases, are included or excluded from the study because of an association with the suspected cause. The use of controls from a respiratory clinic in a study of smoking and bladder cancer has already been cited as an example of this kind of bias.

There are no simple rules that enable bias to be excluded from the design of a study; nor, indeed, is exclusion of all biases always feasible. Suffice it to say that the first step in interpreting an association, or the lack of one, must be assessment of the likely contribution of bias. This assessment may be facilitated if control groups have been selected from two or more sources, for example hospital patients and general practice registers.

Significance tests, which are discussed further on page 92, are used to help resolve the dilemma of whether a particular set of observations is a chance finding. The association shown in Table 5.1 could merely reflect some vagary of sampling, by means of which this particular group of patients and controls happened to differ in their exposure to oestrogens, in which event observations on different patient and control groups are unlikely to reproduce this finding.

Irrespective of the outcome of significance tests, the susceptibility of analytic studies, especially case-control studies, to bias means that great importance can rarely be attached to the results of a single study. Firm conclusions usually rest on two or more studies carried out in different demographic settings. Although some of the case-control studies on smoking and lung cancer are open to criticism because of the method of selection of controls or cases, their results provide strong evidence of the association because they consistently showed higher smoking rates in the cases than controls, even though the magnitude of the difference varied from study to study.

To establish a causal relationship is difficult unless some sound theoretical link exists or can be postulated to explain the observations. In general terms, when data suggest that two variables (or attributes) A and B are associated the possible explanations are (1) A causes B, (2) B causes A, (3) A and B are each determined by some common variables, or (4) some combination of these explanations. The association between water softness and increased cardiovascular mortality rates has been intensively studied for more than a decade. It remains unknown whether some component of drinking water, through its presence or absence, contributes directly to death, or whether both soft water and cardiovascular mortality are independently associated with some other variable such as rainfall. Rain-water is soft, and areas with high rainfall generally use surface water supplies: high rainfall could have some indirect climatic or socio-economic association with cardiovascular mortality.

An association is more likely to be causal if it is:

1. *Strong*. The risk of myocardial infarction in 40-year-old men is increased more than 5-fold in heavy smokers: unrecognized confounding variables are unlikely to account for so large an effect.

2. *Graded*. Threshold effects are uncommon: true causes usually show a continuous dose-response relationship (though it need not be linear).

3. *Independent.* Standardization for possible confounding variables should not abolish a causal association.

4. *Consistent.* The world is complex, and epidemiological surveys are often more difficult to interpret than laboratory experiments. As association is more convincing if it is consistently present in different types of study and in various study populations.

5. *Reversible.* Unless irreversible structural injury has already occurred then abatement of exposure should lead to abatement of risk. Thus users of oral contraceptives lose their special risk of venous thromboembolism within a week or two of stopping 'the pill'.

6. *Plausible.* When John Snow advised dismantling the Broad Street pump he knew nothing of bacteria; acceptance of his story would have been more likely if he could have suggested a possible mechanism, supported by laboratory studies.

The statistical methods of analysis of case-control studies are complex and beyond the scope of this book. It is wise to seek expert guidance. The complexity arises from problems such as the need to take account of paired matching or interactions (see p. 93). The outcome of the analysis will include calculation of the relative risk — if a presumed causal association has been found. If the cases were identified by an initial incidence or prevalence study of a defined population then it will be possible to calculate absolute as well as relative risk, for example the actual incidence of breast cancer according to marital status.

Correlation

Two variables are *correlated* when an increase or decrease in one is associated with an increase or decrease in the other. Figure 5.2, an example of a *scatter diagram*, shows the relation between maternal mortality in England and Wales during 1911–14 and death rates from stroke in the generation born around that time. Areas with higher maternal mortality, whether large towns, administrative counties or London boroughs, have higher stroke rates. This could mean that poor health and physique of mothers is a determinant of the risk of stroke among their offspring. Figure 5.2 shows a *positive correlation* which may be quantified by calculation of the *correlation coefficient* This coefficient is used when inspection of the data on a scatter diagram shows that the relationship between the two variables is adequately described by

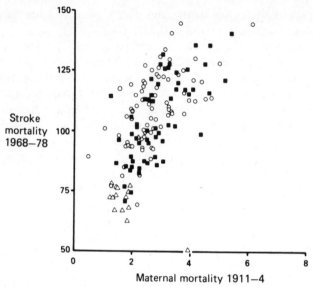

Fig. 5.2 Maternal mortality in 1911–14 and mortality from stroke in 1968–78 in England and Wales. △ = London borough; ○ = County borough; ■ = Administrative centre.

a straight line. Its value ranges between +1 and –1, being zero if the variables are independent. For the data in Figure 5.2 the correlation coefficient is 0.65. Correlations, being one form of association, pose similar problems of interpretation.

Significance tests

As already mentioned, one possible explanation of an association such as that found between endometrial carcinoma and oestrogen therapy is sampling variation. By relating the magnitude of an observed difference, such as that between patients and controls in Table 5.1, to the number of subjects, significance tests (such as the χ^2 test) quantify the frequency with which the observed difference, or a larger one, would occur in a series of samples comprising that particular number of subjects drawn from a population in which exposure to oestrogens and endometrial carcinoma were unrelated. The value of χ^2 for Table 5.1 gives a probability (*P* value) of less than 0.001. This indicates that the difference observed between patients and controls, or a larger difference, would occur on average in less than 1 of every 1000 samples of that size drawn from a population in which endometrial carcinoma and oestrogen therapy were unrelated. The investigator may conclude that the results are more likely to result from a real association between endometrial carcinoma and oestrogen therapy. By convention if P is less than 0.05 the results are often said to be 'statistically significant', supporting, although in no way proving, a real association rather than one due to chance factors in selection of the patients and controls.

The magnitude of a P value depends on both the extent of the difference observed and the number of observations made. Therefore through small numbers of observations it is possible to record a P value that is barely significant, or even not significant at all, despite the fact that the difference observed is large. Conversely through large numbers of observations small differences may achieve statistical significance. This point is clearly important to epidemiologists, whose concern is mainly with those causes of disease that make an important contribution to disease frequency, and whose manipulation offers the possibility of worthwhile preventive action.

Tests for statistical significance may be less widely used in future. Examination of data in relation to a statistical 'null' hypothesis, and the resulting dichotomy into 'significant' or 'non-significant', is less useful than estimates of the size of differences between populations. The difference in mean values (or another summary statistic) of a variable found in two or more groups is an estimate of the result that would have been obtained had all the eligible subjects (the 'population') been examined. Sampling variation makes this estimate imprecise. *Confidence intervals* can be used to summarize this lack of precision. The confidence interval for a difference specifies the range of values that would be plausible were the populations themselves to be compared. Usually a 95% confidence interval is calculated. This defines the range that has a 95% chance of including the population difference. Other intervals (usually 99%) which are wider or narrower (90%) may be calculated. The width of a confidence interval depends on the degree of confidence required, the sample size and the variability of the measurement.

Interactions of causes

Table 5.2 shows the risks of lung cancer occurring 20 or more years after first exposure to asbestos. Among people who did not smoke cigarettes the death rate was 47 per 100 000 person-years

Table 5.2 Excess death rates (per 100 000 person-years) for lung cancer among people exposed to asbestos, according to smoking habits

	Non-smokers	Smokers
Asbestos		
Not exposed	—	111
Exposed	47	590

higher than that in people who were not exposed. Among smokers the death rates in excess of that in non-smokers, who were not exposed and exposed were 111 and 590, respectively. Therefore the combination of asbestos exposure and smoking led to multiplication of their separate risks. This multiplicative increase in risk is an example of interaction of causative influences, whereby one influence modifies the strength of another.

Experimental studies

The results of descriptive and analytic studies rarely incriminate a suspected causal factor to the extent that immediate action to remove or control it in the environment is justified. Among additional kinds of evidence that may be brought to bear are the results of some form of experiment. This subject is discussed in the next chapter (p. 104).

Causes of disease in populations and individuals

Aetiological studies seek to answer two distinct questions. What determines the overall incidence of disease in a population? And what determines which particular individuals within a population fall sick?

Consider, for example, the question 'What causes hypertension?' Research has been largely concerned with explaining why some individuals develop high blood pressure, with interest centering around such matters as genetic factors, salt sensitivity, or activity of the sympathetic system. Figure 5.3 suggests that such reasons for individual susceptibility may be irrelevant to the question of why hypertension is common in some populations yet virtually absent in others. In Kenyan nomads there is almost as much variation between individual blood pressures as there is in a western population, and no doubt there are similar explanations of why some people are at the top end of the distribution. But the reason why hypertension is absent in one population and prevalent

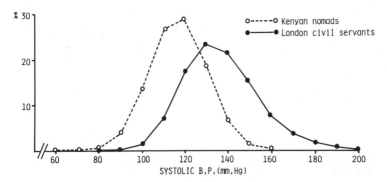

Fig. 5.3 Distribution of systolic blood pressure in Kenyan nomads and London civil servants.

in another must lie in some mass characteristic, perhaps dietary, which has elevated the whole distribution.

The determinants of individual susceptibility reflect the intrinsic variability of individual behaviour and genetic constitution. Differences in incidence between populations usually reflect mass characteristics, either environmental or behavioural. The distinction is vital to preventive strategy: mass diseases have mass causes, and so their prevention calls for a mass approach.

Population attributable risk

The importance of a health hazard to a population depends both on the size of the risk for exposed individuals and on the prevalence of exposure. The product of these two factors is the *population attributable risk*. If a risk is uncommon (for example, exposure to large amounts of wood dust in the furniture industry) then the disease (nasal cancer) constitutes only a small community risk, however serious it may be to the individuals involved. On the other hand a risk may be individually so small as to be disregarded, yet if it is common it can cause a great many cases. This may be illustrated by Down's syndrome in relation to maternal age (Table 5.3). Below the age of 30 years the risk to the individual is tiny; yet because most births occur in this age group, it yields a half of all the cases of Down's syndrome. As commonly occurs, many people exposed to a small risk yield more cases than a few people exposed to a large risk.

The population attributable risk provides a measure of the potential impact of an effective control measure. From Table 5.3

Table 5.3   The risk of Down's syndrome according to maternal age*

Maternal age (years)	Risk of Down's syndrome per 1000 births	No. births in age group as % of all births	No. cases of Down's syndrome in age group as % of all cases
<30	0.7	78	51
30–34	1.3	16	20
35–39	3.7	5	16
40–44	13.1	0.95	11
≥45	34.6	0.05	2
All ages	1.5	100	100

* Alberman E, Berry C 1979 Community Medicine 1: 89

it follows that a plan for screening and selective abortion offered to all women over the age of 35 years could not hope to reduce Down's syndrome births by more than 29%.

In summary, there are three ways of expressing a causal risk, each appropriate to a quite different situation. If a = the incidence of disease in those exposed, b = incidence in non-exposed, and p = prevalence of exposure, then:

Relative risk $= a/b$ estimates the strength of a cause

Excess (attributable risk) $= (a - b)$ indicates an individual's need for preventive action

Population attributable risk $= (a - b) \times p$ indicates the population's need for preventive action

6. Evaluation of preventive measures

The practical application of aetiology is an attempt to prevent disease. This may involve an attack on the primary agent, as in the prophylaxis of bacterial endocarditis by antibiotic administration before dental procedures. Transmission of the primary agent may be interrupted as when radioactive emissions from nuclear plants are reduced. When an environmental hazard cannot be removed it may be possible to protect the individual against it, as by encouraging noise-exposed workers to wear ear plugs or muffs. The individual's resistance can be raised, by immunization against infectious diseases, for example, or by nutritional improvement in populations where malnutrition increases susceptibility to tuberculosis.

The prevention of an acute infectious disease is conceptually simple, since the aim is to prevent the entire illness. With chronic diseases, however, one may distinguish between measures to prevent the first onset of illness (*primary prevention*) and measures aimed against progression or recurrences (*secondary prevention*). This distinction is often not clear-cut since the underlying disease process may be present for years before clinical illness is apparent. Autopsy studies of seemingly normal areas of bronchial mucosa have given the results shown in Table 6.1. Evidently the lungs of most cigarette smokers contain multiple foci of premalignant metaplasia, and 8% of sections even showed in situ carcinoma. Such lesions were much less frequent in the lungs of ex-smokers. This suggests that cessation of smoking leads to regression of established early disease rather than to primary prevention. In practice it may be more relevant to categorize as 'primary prevention' those measures that are applied to individuals in whom disease is not yet clinically recognized, and as 'secondary prevention' those measures taken to reduce the risk of a second

Table 6.1 The association between cigarette smoking and the presence of premalignant bronchial changes in routine autopsy sections (groups matched for age, sex, residence and occupation)*

| Smoking group | Epithelial metaplasia | % of sections showing lesion | |
		Atypical nuclei	In situ carcinoma
Non-smokers	25	1	0
Ex-smokers	67	6	1
Continuing smokers	98	81	8

* Auerbach O et al (1962) New England Journal of Medicine 267: 111

attack. Screening in order to achieve earlier diagnosis can be considered as an activity intermediate between primary and secondary prevention.

Need for objective evidence of effectiveness

In clinical medicine it is the patient who takes the initiative in seeking help from the doctor. By contrast in preventive medicine the initiative comes from doctors. This imposes on them a special responsibility to justify their intrusion.

When measures are hygienic, such as addition of aluminium or fluoride to water, it may be impossible to seek consent from individual recipients: all must have it, or none. Furthermore it is often only a small minority who will actually receive any benefit. In England in 1968 it was estimated that 750 children needed to receive BCG vaccination in order to prevent one notified case of tuberculosis; 10 years later this number had risen to 3000. Decisions on medical management depend on balancing the benefits against the costs or hazards. In the clinical field every patient has a complaint and hopes for an early benefit from therapy; in the preventive field only some will benefit, yet all must be exposed to the procedure.

Before a preventive measure is adopted it is important to obtain an objective and quantitative prediction of benefits and losses; for once a service has become accepted its subsequent evaluation or possible withdrawal are likely to meet opposition from public conservatism and vested medical interests, as the following examples suggest.

Examples of unsubstantiated measures

For many years powdered iron was added to flour in the belief that it helped to prevent iron-deficiency anaemia and hence make people in some way fitter. A randomized controlled trial in the 1960s showed that unfortunately this form of iron was not absorbed, and haemoglobin levels were indistinguishable in groups receiving fortified and unfortified bread. Furthermore the treatment of mild or moderate iron-deficiency anaemia by more effective means did not lead to any detectable improvement in symptoms or 'fitness'. However, powdered iron continued to be added to bread.

When Almroth Wright introduced his phenol-preserved typhoid vaccine it was used with apparent success among the troops in the First World War. Subsequently an alternative alcohol-preserved vaccine was introduced, because tests in laboratory animals showed that this was more effective as indicated by the rise in titre of Vi-antibody. Throughout the Second World War the new vaccine was the accepted standard and hundreds of thousands of doses were administered. It was many years later that randomized controlled trials in Yugoslavia demonstrated that, contrary to laboratory evidence and established practice, the alcohol-preserved vaccine was less than half as effective in preventing human typhoid fever as the old phenol-preserved variety introduced by Almroth Wright.

At a more mundane level one may ponder the countless Britons who have shivered through the winter with train or office windows open, in the not unreasonable hope that this would make them less liable to catch their neighbour's cold. The hypothesis unfortunately has not survived objective scientific evaluation. In a controlled experiment forced ventilation was introduced in one-half of a series of offices, and attack rates of coryza were recorded. No differences emerged, either in this experiment or in others where the investigators studied the effects of a hexylresorcinol spray or of ultraviolet irradiation of the air.

Types of evidence

These examples all point to the same conclusion: evidence for the effectiveness of a preventive measure needs to be direct, not indirect or merely theoretical, and it should be obtained before a routine service is introduced. The evidence may take various forms:

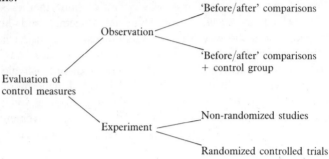

Observational studies

In the cholera epidemic of 1854 John Snow managed to convince the authorities that the pump in Broad Street, Soho was the source of a severe local outbreak and should be dismantled. This and similar evidence led to effective control of London's water supplies, and cholera ceased to be a mass problem. More recent examples of this kind include the dramatic and almost complete disappearance of paralytic poliomyelitis in many countries after vaccination was introduced, and the decline in deaths from lung cancer following control of high-tar cigarettes.

These examples point to the requirements for drawing confident conclusions about preventive measures from a 'before/after' comparison of disease rates. There must be adequate information on incidence and diagnostic practices before the change is introduced. There must be a single change in relevant conditions; its adoption must be simultaneous and widespread; and its effectiveness in preventing the disease must be large and rapid.

In some current examples of before/after comparisons these requirements have not been met. The true impact of screening for cervical cancer remains uncertain because the procedure has been adopted incompletely and over a period of years, because it is less than completely effective, and because the incidence of the disease was declining before screening was commenced.

Figure 6.1 shows the remarkable recent decline in mortality from stroke in Australia. An obvious explanation for this is the widespread use of antihypertensive drugs, but there are reasons for thinking that much of the change is unrelated to therapy. The decline began before the widespread use of antihypertensive drugs,

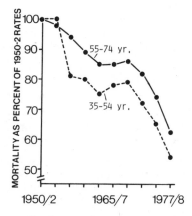

Fig. 6.1 Declining mortality from cerebrovascular accidents among men in Australia from 1950 to 1978 (three-year average rates).

and it included the older age groups among whom antihypertensive therapy was not so widely used; however, around 1970, coinciding with widespread use of more potent drugs, there was a clear acceleration of the decline.

Control groups

There was once a study to determine whether an autogenous respiratory bacterial vaccine would confer protection against the common cold. Volunteer medical students were asked to record how many colds they had experienced in the previous winter. The average was 5.6. They were then given the vaccine in the autumn, and in the following winter they experienced on average only 1.8 colds each: a seeming success for the vaccine. However, half of them had in fact received only a placebo, and the full results are shown in Table 6.2. The improvement in the vaccine group is matched by equally striking improvement among control subjects: evidently students tended to volunteer for the trial because of an unusually bad experience in the previous

Table 6.2 Results of a trial of an autogenous vaccine against the common cold

	Average no. of winter colds	
	Pre-treatment	Post-treatment
Vaccine group	5.6	1.8
Control group	5.5	1.7

winter. In many conditions a bad period tends to be followed by an improvement, just as a remission may be followed by an exacerbation. This is an example of the statistical phenomenon known as *regression to the mean*, which is the tendency for abnormally high values to be followed by more average (that is lower) values, and vice versa. This phenomenon ('the physician's friend') operates in newly detected cases of any condition that fluctuates in severity, whether this is the common cold, backache, hypertension, or some biochemical deviation from the normal range. Since patients are more likely to seek help or to be given treatment during an exacerbation, regression to the mean makes it difficult to separate the effects of intervention from a natural trend towards improvement. A control group makes such a distinction possible.

The ideal control group is selected by a process of random allocation, as in the previous example, and trials of this type will be considered in detail later. Less satisfactory, but more frequent and often much simpler, are studies that utilize some natural comparison group. For example, in early studies of perinatal mortality the rates among the babies of three groups of primigravidae in Aberdeen, those in a private nursing home, a less expensive nursing home, and the city's maternity hospital, were compared. This gave an immediate insight into the inverse relation between perinatal mortality and maternal stature; and hence showed the potential importance of improving the nutrition and health of young women in preventing perinatal death.

Preventive measures may be environmental, such as fluoride in the water supply, or personal, such as vaccination or change in personal habits. In the absence of results from controlled trials the benefits from personal measures may be assessed by comparing the experiences of those who change and those who do not, although it has to be assumed that those who adopt the measure would otherwise have been subject to the same risks of disease as those who do not. Sometimes this assumption is manifestly not true. For example, some groups of people who have recently stopped smoking have shown a higher mortality from cardio-respiratory disorders than those who continue to smoke. Obviously this does not prove that it is dangerous to stop smoking: it probably means that many who change their habits do so because of incipient ill health.

The babies of mothers who stop smoking during pregnancy tend to resemble in birth-weight those of non-smokers rather than those whose mothers continue to smoke. However, a mother who chooses to give up smoking during pregnancy may well have smoked less and inhaled less than one who continues, and this, rather than the fact of cessation, could account for the more favourable outcome. This example again emphasizes the need in non-randomized studies to question whether the study and control groups are truly comparable.

The evaluation of preventive measures has largely depended on critical assessment of imperfectly controlled experiments. This approach is crude and liable to various kinds of bias. Unless the observed change in rates is large, it is always possible that it may be no more than a misleading coincidence. In the past the consequences of error would often not have been serious, for three reasons. Firstly, preventive measures commonly involved removal of a noxious factor (pollution of water or air, or cigarette smoking) rather than the addition of some new factor. Secondly, where prevention was by positive measures (such as immunization), these were usually introduced in order to control common or serious diseases. Finally, the measures were often cheap and caused relatively little disturbance to the recipients.

The kinds of preventive measure debated today often differ in each of these respects. The measure may involve exposure to some substance such as cholesterol-lowering drugs or post-menopausal oestrogens, whose long-term toxic effects cannot be known with certainty. Toxic hazards are a more serious cause for concern when the disease to be prevented is uncommon. For instance, the risks of immunization against whooping cough were relatively unimportant when the disease itself killed many children, but they led to a questioning of the policy of mass vaccination when it was claimed (probably wrongly) that serious complications of the procedure outnumbered deaths from the disease. This reassessment was possible because the complications of immunization are acute and generally obvious; but other hazards are less easily assessed, for example those of mass drug treatment of hypercholesterolaemia.

Health services should optimize the benefits obtainable from limited resources, and this requires measurement of costs and benefits. Costs of modern medical services can be large, as with mass screening for breast cancer or for rare congenital amino-acidurias, and correspondingly stronger evidence is needed to justify their introduction. These considerations lie behind the advocacy of randomized controlled trials in the evaluation of preventive as well as therapeutic services. It is true that preventive trials can be major undertakings, but nevertheless even the large costs of the recent Swedish trial of breast cancer screening were small in relation to the medical and human costs of a wrong decision. The essential point is that major services ought not to be launched without adequate justification, even when this requires a full-scale controlled preventive trial.

Experimental studies

Aims

In the experimental evaluation of a preventive programme three questions need to be answered.

1. *How much will it benefit the community?* This depends not only on the inherent effectiveness of the measure, but also on the level of its acceptance by the community (*adherence* or *compliance*). In a trial the combined outcome of effectiveness and compliance is measured by the difference in incidence of the disorder between the intervention and control groups. In preventive trials of drugs (e.g. in hypertension or in the prevention of 'traveller's diarrhoea') or of health education (e.g. diet in relation to coronary heart disease or the effects of smoking cessation), the size of the community benefit may be much less than the theoretical prediction, simply because many people do not take their tablets or do as they are advised.

2. *What are its risks to the recipients?* These comprise the immediate hazards, such as anaphylaxis following pollen injections to control hay fever, and long-term effects, whose detection may pose formidable practical difficulties.

3. *What will be the costs to medical resources in money and work-load?*

A good trial should provide a quantitative answer to each of these questions, since a final decision to institute a preventive programme involves balancing of all gains and losses.

Selection of the experimental population

The subjects in the study sample should adequately represent the reference population to which the measure, if successful, will be applied. For example, they should be similar as regards the incidence of the disease to be prevented. This was achieved in the Medical Research Council trial of pertussis immunization by studying children from state schools and by obtaining a high response rate. By contrast it may be unwise to assume that the results of trials of coronary artery surgery in the secondary prevention of coronary heart disease, carried out in leading centres, are a sound guide to its wider application.

Advantages of randomized allocation

As in a therapeutic trial, the final decision on a subject's acceptance into the trial must be made without knowledge of the group to which he or she will be allocated. As a further device to preclude bias this allocation should be randomly determined (see p. 42). Randomization is the hallmark of an honest trial, and a study in which the investigator retained any control over the allocation of the subjects should be viewed with grave suspicion.

Normally the allocation to intervention or control status is determined for individual subjects one at a time, for example to receive vaccine or placebo. However, if the test measure involves either environmental manipulation, such as fluoridation of water, or community health education, as in control of gonorrhoea, it will be necessary to allocate communities rather than individuals. Thus in the WHO European coronary heart disease prevention trial, participating factories were allocated randomly to intervention or control status. Individuals in the former were screened for coronary risk factors and given health education, whereas the control factories were left alone.

Checking initial comparability

Relevant characteristics of the intervention and control groups must be compared in order to test the effectiveness of randomization: it is necessary to ensure that important differences have not occurred, albeit by chance, in factors that may affect the incidence of disease.

Management of control group

This should be so far as possible identical with the management of the intervention group in all respects except the experimental measure. In order to achieve this in circumstances where the same medical team provides care for both groups a 'double-blind' design may be necessary. In other trials the comparison may be between an intervention group managed by the research team and a 'usual care' group managed by the ordinary medical services. In a controlled trial among civil servants of the effectiveness of antismoking advice an initial screening examination identified those cigarette smokers who had risk factors for cardiorespiratory disease, and a randomly selected half of these men were referred to a special advisory team. It would have been unethical to deny control subjects any access to medical advice and they were referred instead to their general practitioners, thus forming a 'usual care' control group.

Assessment of outcome

Outcome may be measured by the occurrence of an event (such as a neonatal death or a recurrence of rheumatic fever), and the results are then analysed in terms of incidence rates; or it may be measured by some change in a quantitative variable (such as body-weight in an obesity study or hearing loss in noise-exposed workers), when results can usually be summarized by their means and standard deviations.

It is insufficient evidence of benefit to show that a particular measure improves the results of laboratory tests. The measures of outcome should wherever possible be those that are directly important to the subjects, that is death, disability or symptoms.

There are two kinds of end-point in a trial, namely *positive* (benefits) and *negative* (complications); both must be measured. For example, in a trial of the effect of antihypertensive drugs on the risk of cardiovascular disease it would be essential to measure not only the incidence of strokes and heart attacks but also the incidence of drug side-effects, together with the effect on 'quality of life' of prolonged medical intervention. All of these are relevant to the final decision on whether the preventive measure should be generally adopted.

In the WHO clofibrate trial the investigators were shocked to find that mortality in the treatment group was one-third higher than in controls, corresponding to an excess of about 1 death per 1000 patient-years. In treating sick patients a risk of this low order might be perfectly acceptable; but in prevention, where each individual has only a small probability of benefit, even a small risk may be critical. Thus in prevention, safety is of paramount importance. Unfortunately it may be impossible to identify small but important long-term risks, and this greatly limits the use of drugs in prevention.

The follow-up and ascertainment of outcome must be equally thorough in the intervention and control groups, with equal and preferably high follow-up rates: it has often been found that default is more likely in those who have not complied with advice or treatment or who have become ill. Similarly it is necessary that the decision on who has suffered an end-point event should be protected from bias. In a 'double-blind' design this is assured by keeping both patient and investigator unaware of the patient's group; otherwise end-points must be determined objectively by the strict application of pre-set rules. When a certain difference in outcome has been observed between the experimental and control groups, the first step in its interpretation is to consider whether it might be due entirely to *bias* introduced through faulty design or execution, particularly in the measurement of outcome. Next its *statistical significance* is considered. Initial randomization will have ensured that at the outset of the trial the only differences between the groups were those due to chance, and it must now be decided how likely it is that chance could also produce a difference in outcome as large as that observed. This is based on calculation of the P value (see p. 92). However, a difference may be statistically significant but practically unimportant: hence the need next to consider its *magnitude*.

Conversely, and more usually, an important effect may fail to achieve statistical significance if the trial is too small.

The conclusions from a negative trial are these. If an effect of practical importance might have escaped detection through small numbers then a larger trial is called for. If compliance was poor then the preventive measure should not be finally abandoned until alternative methods have been explored for its more effective delivery; but in the meantime it should not be implemented. If compliance was adequate and the trial size large enough to exclude a useful benefit, then the measure is inherently useless.

Implementing results

The decision on whether or not to adopt a particular medical policy depends on balancing the benefits and costs of the alternatives. This is not easy, particularly when disturbance and morbidity associated with a preventive measure have to be set against a reduction of mortality from the disease. The *costing* of a preventive programme can also be difficult. One component which tends to be overlooked is the amount of time demanded, both from the medical team and from the subjects themselves. It is also necessary to consider the effects of diverting scarce skills from other and perhaps more fruitful applications. The advantage of the controlled trial is that it represents the best means available of getting the quantitative estimates that are necessary for rational decisions. The data, however, do not make the decision; that requires a judgement of the values to be assigned to the various benefits and costs.

Trials to test aetiological hypotheses

Evidence on causation given by descriptive and analytic studies is often inconclusive. Sometimes it is possible to strengthen it by conducting an experiment. Semelweiss, a 19th century obstetrician, drew attention to the higher incidence of puerperal fever among women delivered by medical students (who attended septic autopsies) as compared with those delivered by midwives. People remained unconvinced of the septic origin of the disease until it was seen that hygienic control measures led to an impressive decline in incidence.

Retrolental fibroplasia was first described in 1942 and soon became recognized in many countries as the leading cause of blindness in children. Descriptive studies quickly demonstrated its close association with oxygen administration to premature babies, but doctors were loth to discontinue a valued therapy. In 1955 they were finally convinced by the results of a large controlled trial (Table 6.3) in which babies with birth-weights of 1500 g or less were allocated to two groups: in one group all babies received

Table 6.3 A trial to study the effect of continuous oxygen therapy on the risk of retrolental fibroplasia*

Grade of disease	% of infants	
	Continuous O_2	Restricted O_2
Nil	28	70
Grades 1–2	48	23
Grade 3+	24	7
Total no. of infants	53	245

* Kinsey V E, Hemphill F M 1955 American Journal of Ophthalmology 40: 166

50% oxygen therapy for 28 days, while in the other group it was used only for clinical emergencies.

Few if any acquired diseases are the outcome of a single cause. The cause may be generally *necessary* (such as a certain level of saturated fat intake in the genesis of coronary heart disease), but not by itself *sufficient*: other factors, both genetic and environmental, influence individual susceptibility or aggravate the disease process. This multifactorial aetiology must be considered both in patient care and in preventive strategy. For example, the proper treatment of a patient with hypertension requires not only drug therapy but attention to other coronary risk factors. And prevention of lung cancer in asbestos workers requires both measures against inhalation of asbestos fibres and avoidance of smoking. Multifactorial aetiology also affects preventive trials, which may be designed to measure the total effect of a package of measures rather than of a single factor by itself.

When a disease appears after a long latent period or is the result of long-continued exposure there are serious difficulties in mounting a trial. Despite control of exposure to antioxidants in the rubber industry cases of bladder cancer continue to occur, presumably because earlier exposure set in motion some irreversible pathological process. It has recently been suggested that genetic damage by radiation, mostly affecting recessive genes, may not be manifest for several generations. Such delayed effects, which could be important, are difficult if not impossible to assess in humans.

A negative outcome to preventive measures does not necessarily disprove that particular aetiology: it may mean only that intervention started too late and that the proper controlled trial would be one that began with young subjects who would be followed for many years. Such a trial is required to test the nature of the relationship between atherosclerotic disease and infant nutrition. Unfortunately few investigators are willing and able to undertake such long-term research.

Epidemiology and patient care

7. Natural history and prognosis

A rational decision on whether or not to give a certain treatment is possible only if the outcome of the disease without treatment is known. Unfortunately such decisions — whether, for example, to treat a patient with mild hypertension or to recommend an elective cholecystectomy in a patient with gallstones — all too often require data that are not available. These data are of course especially difficult to acquire for diseases with a high fatality where doctors feel compelled to act in an attempt to save life. It is not known whether the poor prognosis following surgical treatment of malignant cerebral glioma would be any worse if surgery were not attempted.

In addition to therapy, an important part of the doctor's task is to give a prognosis to patients or their relatives. This again requires knowledge of the natural history of the disease and the way in which it may be modified by special features of a particular case, and by treatment. For many of the chronic and incurable disorders that now dominate medical practice there are insufficient data to enable the doctor to give useful prognoses. Psychiatrists, for example, are much handicapped by inadequate knowledge of the outcome of chronic mental illness.

Clinical experience cannot, by itself, provide an adequate guide to progress and outcome. There are two principle reasons for this: the biases involved in case selection, and incomplete follow-up of patients. The purpose of this chapter is to suggest how epidemiological data may usefully supplement clinical data.

Limitations of clinical experience

Case selection

For many diseases, the cases seen by any one doctor are a highly unrepresentative group of all cases in the community, brought to the doctor's attention by a variety of selective factors. Severity is one such factor. Surveys have shown that many patients with peptic ulcer do not consult a doctor. Among those who come to the general practitioner, the usual course (as revealed by a study of the natural history of peptic ulcer in general practice over a 15-year period) is an initial phase with frequent episodes of disabling pain. This reaches a peak after 5–10 years and is followed by progressive remission and usually complete recovery. However, in hospital wards the picture is of life-threatening emergencies due to haemorrhage or perforation.

In addition to the severity of the disease, the likelihood of a patient receiving medical attention is influenced by the occurrence of symptoms and tolerance of them, access to the doctor and to diagnostic facilities, and by medical interest in the condition and its treatment. Coronary heart disease is more likely to be diagnosed in business executives who worry about minor pains in the chest or who undergo an annual electrocardiographic check-up. Deafness or visual disturbance is less likely to be recognized in an old person, or depression in those who live alone. Patients diagnosed as having urinary tract infection tend to have symptoms and often have structural abnormalities of the renal tract. In contrast, population surveys have shown that as many as 2% of schoolgirls have bacteriuria, but this is usually asymptomatic and undiagnosed and in about 80% of these cases the renal tract is normal on imaging.

As a result of such selective factors the cases of a disease that come to medical attention represent a biased sample. There tends to be over-representation of chronic and severe cases, patients with lower symptom thresholds, and those with 'interesting' medical or social features; and there tends to be under-representation of rapid deaths, the milder or spontaneously recovering cases, the stoical and the old. As a result the hospital picture of a disease and its course can be grossly distorted or incomplete.

The effects of case selection in hospital practice may be compounded by the dispersion of cases with the same disease among different specialities. Giant cell arteritis, for example, may be under the care of neurologists, ophthalmologists, general physicians, geriatricians or rheumatologists. The personal experience of any one specialist must necessarily be an inadequate guide to prognosis.

Clinical case selection not only influences our view of the natural history of disease: it may also lead to false deductions about the association between one disorder and another, or between a disorder and the characteristics of patients.

Prevalence surveys in the population show no association between migraine and social class, yet in clinical series there tends to be an over-representation of social class 1 and 2. Presumably this is due to their different use of medical care facilities. The effect of such bias in ascertainment may be to suggest false associations, in this instance between migraine and social class. In this way medical myths may originate, and once established a myth tends to be self-perpetuating. Doctors have been led to believe that mild anaemia causes tiredness. As a result they are more likely to measure the haemoglobin if a patient complains of lassitude, and thus anaemia is more likely to be discovered in those who feel tired. Epistaxis is widely thought to be an important complication of hypertension. Patients with nose-bleeds are thus more likely to have their blood pressures measured, and an association between *diagnosed* hypertension and epistaxis is thereby confirmed. However, population studies have shown that hypertension is associated with little increase in the incidence of epistaxis, and most nose-bleeds in hypertensives are unrelated to this disorder.

Any imaginative doctor with access to sufficient clinical material can earn fame by describing a new syndrome: he or she has only to write up several cases each showing the same association of distinctive features. In this way Drs Paterson, Kelly, Plummer and Vinson have all acquired medical immortality by describing a syndrome of iron-deficiency anaemia, dysphagia, and postcricoid 'web'. It is not in question that such cases exist; but so also do cases of each of the three separate components of the syndrome, as well as each of the three possible pairs. In a population survey of these three individual conditions, no evidence was found that the 'syndrome' of all three in the same person occurred any more often than would be expected from the chance association of three unrelated conditions.

This example should not disparage the clinical impression. The astute observation of previously unsuspected associations is the origin of much new knowledge. The conclusion to draw is that clinical impressions need to be tested objectively, and one way of doing this may be an epidemiological study.

Incomplete follow-up

A neurologist's view of multiple sclerosis tends to be unduly gloomy. The one-third of patients in whom the disease remits without residual disability do not continue to attend the clinic. Those in whom the disease runs a less favourable course return again and again.

An ENT surgeon was heard to say to a patient, 'And if you have any more trouble, come back and I'll wash out your sinuses again'. One may wonder whether he was confusing the deterrent quality of his treatment with its effectiveness. The experience of many doctors treating hypertension is that in time the side-effects of drugs tend to wear off, and blood pressure control is more satisfactory among patients who have been attending the clinic for a long time. This encouraging impression may be due largely to the tendency of patients experiencing side-effects to default, whereas those who comply with the doctor's advice and treatment continue to attend.

The clinical follow-up study

Since clinical experience on its own is an insufficient guide to the outcome of diseases in which progression is slow and the outcome variable, it must be supplemented by other data. The clinical follow-up study is one way in which additional data may be obtained. Such studies are not strictly epidemiological, since the findings cannot usually be related to a defined whole community. Nevertheless the method of follow-up enquiry usually involves an approach to the community, and the techniques used for all group studies are akin to those of epidemiological surveys.

Soon after the introduction of radio-iodine therapy for thyrotoxicosis it became apparent that in some cases it was followed within a year or so by the onset of hypothyroidism. A follow-up study was urgently required to determine the frequency of this serious complication and ways in which it could be avoided.

The ideal study in this situation would be one planned prospectively. Diagnostic criteria, methods of investigation and record forms can be designed in advance, and complete and uniform data may be assembled. However, when the questions to be studied relate to long-term complications the delay involved in a prospectively planned enquiry may be unacceptable, and it becomes necessary to attempt the frustrating task of searching the archives and carrying out a retrospective follow-up. Several such studies were carried out on thyrotoxic patients treated with radio-iodine, and they showed that between 2 and 5% of these patients became hypothyroid each year.

When carrying out retrospective follow-up studies certain points have to be borne in mind.

Case definition and ascertainment

It is rarely easy to define what is meant by 'a case', even of a well-known disease (see p. 30). In follow-up studies particular problems arise from atypical, borderline and confirmed cases, and it is important to define rigid diagnostic criteria at the outset of the study, even though they may be arbitrary. The follow-up should include all *new* cases first seen in some defined time period, for if all cases under care are included, both old and new, the study is biased towards surviving and more chronic cases. Since the purpose of any scientific enquiry is to produce generalizable results it is important to define selection factors that may have influenced referral, hospital admission and diagnosis of the cases, including if possible some check on the veracity of the diagnostic register or other method by which cases were ascertained.

Pilot study

It is wise to make an initial study of a small sample of records, to determine approximately how many cases there are likely to be, what proportion of notes have been lost, and how much essential information was not recorded. This sample may also be used to test how many patients can no longer be traced. Pilot studies are a prudent precaution against large-scale disaster.

Record design

Relevant information will be extracted from clinical records and transferred to a special data sheet, which should be designed to facilitate later retrieval and analysis. The method of analysis should therefore be decided at the outset. Often it is convenient to precode the initial data sheet, laying it out in such a way that computer entry (if this form of analysis is to be used) can be done directly without the need for an intermediary transfer sheet.

Follow-up

When the patients have been identified and base-line information recorded, the follow up commences. (The problems of follow-up have been considered in Chapter 3, in the section on longitudinal studies.) It may be easy to obtain follow-up information on the first 80% or so of patients simply by writing to them at their last known home address, but higher follow-up rates are usually essential (p. 44). A study was undertaken of the 624 patients with ulcerative colitis treated at Oxford. Follow-up information was obtained from 100% and the findings on relapse rates, cancer incidence and mortality are therefore trustworthy. If the follow-up had included only 90%, the unseen 10% might well have contained a disproportionate number of cases with a bad outcome.

In order to achieve a high follow-up rate it is usually necessary to use more than one method. Possible methods include home visits, a search of central death certificates, social security records, employment pension records, and the NHS central records or local general practice lists.

Methods of describing prognosis

Case fatality ratio

The case fatality ratio (CFR) is the usual clinical measure of mortality. (An operative mortality rate is a special form of CFR.) The CFR is defined as the proportion of illness episodes ending fatally:

$$\text{Case fatality ratio \%} = \frac{\text{No. dying in episode}}{\text{Total no. of patient episodes}} \times 100$$

The CFR differs from the epidemiological measure of mortality, the mortality rate, in respect of both the numerator and the denominator. In the mortality rate the numerator is the number of persons dying from the condition within a specified time period, such as a year, but the numerator for the CFR is the number of patients dying in the particular episode of illness, such as a hospital admission for haematemesis. This can raise difficulties since the definition of the illness episode is not a specific period of time. Often it refers to the period of medical care, as in a coronary care unit. In this case the CFR tends to be lower in situations where earlier discharge is practised, and the experience of different units can be compared only if they have adopted the same criterion of duration for estimating the CFR or if the lengths of stay in each unit have the same distribution.

The denominator for a mortality rate is a related community comprising sick and well persons, whereas for a CFR the denominator is the number of illness episodes observed during a particular period.

When comparing the prognosis of different groups of patients it is essential to take into account differences in their age and sex structure, together with factors influencing initial case selection. Thus it is meaningless to report the crude (all-ages) CFR for myocardial infarction in a particular unit: interpretation is not possible unless the comparison takes account of age, severity and length of stay.

Survival rates

The case fatality rate is only an appropriate measure of outcome for a short-term risk, since the period considered is that of an acute episode of illness. To measure the outcome over a longer period of time, for example among cancer patients, it is more appropriate to use survival rates, in which any convenient time period may be specified; for example:

$$5\text{-year survival rate} = \frac{\text{Total no. of patients alive after 5 years}}{\text{Total no. of patients diagnosed (or treated)}}$$

As with the CFR, the age and sex distribution of the patients needs to be specified.

If the follow-up period is long then the survival rate will reflect not only deaths due to the disease in question but also those due to the general causes of mortality in the population. Provided that the age-specific mortality rates for the general population are available it is possible to make an appropriate allowance for this attrition, yielding what is known as a *relative survival rate*. (For example, the relative 5-year survival rate for prostatic cancer in England and Wales is 36%, compared with a crude rate of 22%.)

The survival period is usually reckoned from the date of diagnosis or the start of treatment, since this is more easily defined than the first onset of the illness. Thus if earlier diagnosis is achieved, as a result of screening for example, the patients' survival will be reckoned from an earlier point in time; as a result the survival rate will appear to improve even if the true total duration of the illness remains unchanged. This *lead time* gained by earlier diagnosis may make it difficult to compare different series of patients, unless the diagnostic processes are known to be the same.

A similar problem arises in assessing the results of earlier treatment or operation. If the disease is one where spontaneous recoveries occur, then earlier surgery may get the credit for cures that would have occurred naturally. On the other hand, as a result of the earlier diagnosis of cancer an increased proportion of tumours may still be resectable. Thus a series with earlier surgery will be adversely weighted with rapidly growing tumours with a bad prognosis, while a series with later diagnosis will exclude such tumours, which will no longer be operable.

By the time that lung cancer is diagnosed the disease is already advanced and prognosis is bad, as illustrated by the experience of a Danish thoracic surgeon (Table 7.1). His honest presentation of results was made possible by a combination of a hospital diagnostic register and a community cancer register; it shows how the apparent prognosis as measured by the survival rate, is affected by the definition of the 'at risk' group. From the viewpoint of the surgeon's follow-up clinic the apparent 5-year survival rate (9%) was 3 times better than the true picture in the community as a whole (3%). These particular results do not reveal the effect of resection on an individual's chance of survival, since it may be that the surgeon is operating on those patients who are likely to do better anyway; but they do put the contribution of surgery into perspective.

Table 7.2 provides some further contrasts, from cancer registry data, of the different survival rates in the community as a whole and in patients treated radically in hospital. At some sites, such as skin and uterus, diagnosis is easy and most tumours are resectable, nearly all cases come to surgery, and the hospital estimate of prognosis is close to the rate for the whole community. For other

Table 7.1 Prognosis of lung cancer in Copenhagen

Group	No. of cases	5-year survival rate %
Resected lung	203	9
Total coming to surgeon	264	7
Total admitted to hospital	516	3.5
All cases (community register)	600	3

Table 7.2 Common cancers: comparison of survival rates for radically treated patients with those for the whole community (data from Birmingham Regional Cancer Register)

Site of cancer	5-year survival rate %	
	Radical treatment	All cases
Uterus (body)	71	62
Skin (squamous cell)	61	58
Breast	52	43
Skin (melanoma)	48	44
Uterus (cervix)	48	40
Colon	41	20
Stomach	15	4
Oesophagus	10	3
Pancreas	8	0.6

sites, such as colon and stomach, many patients never come to operation and so surgical experience yields an estimate that is much too optimistic.

Life-table analysis

The simple survival rate has two limitations as a measure of prognosis for life: it fails to distinguish early and late deaths, and it wastes the information that may be available for patients who have been followed for less than the whole period.

In an ideal study all patients would have been followed up for the same length of time and there would be no patients whose fate is unknown. In reality patients are diagnosed and enter the study at various times and in some there is incomplete follow-up, so that the period of observation varies from one patient to another. A life-table analysis deals with this problem by estimating survival rates independently for each of a series of intervals calculated from the start of treatment. For each interval it is first necessary to define the appropriate group for that particular part of the analysis, comprising only those patients (living or dead) who have been in the study for that time from the start of treatment; the survival rate for the period is then expressed as the proportion of these patients who are alive at its end (with a small correction for those lost to follow-up during the period). This method makes the fullest use of all the available information: a patient who entered the study only one year previously, or one who was lost

Table 7.3 Life-table analysis of kidney graft survival according to matching for HLA tissue types

Months from transplantation	Good match		Poor match	
	No. in study at start of period	% surviving period	No. in study at start of period	% surviving period
1	47	87	271	71
3	39	76	191	53
6	34	74	139	45
12	32	62	113	41
18	26	60	102	37

to follow-up after one year, will not be altogether excluded from analysis but will contribute to the one-year results.

Table 7.3 provides an example of a life-table analysis of the results of a renal transplant programme. The effect of good matching on outcome is estimated optimally for each stage of follow-up, even though only a minority of patients had completed the whole period.

Record linkage

Record linkage, which is discussed on page 25, offers another method by which clinical information on prognosis may be supplemented. If the various patients' records that are routinely compiled were linked together this would give a fuller picture of the course of an illness and of different illnesses occurring in the life of an individual. From even such simple developments of record linkage as the matching of hospital discharge and mortality data much needed data on prognosis would at once become available.

The Office of Population Censuses and Surveys for England and Wales has instituted a longitudinal study that links the census data from a 1% random sample of the population with subsequent birth and health records. One of its remarkable findings is that mortality is 25% higher in men living in local authority rented accommodation than in those who own their own homes.

The precursor and preclinical phases of disease

The results shown in Table 7.4 are taken from a 2-year follow-up of patients discharged from a general medical ward. The finding

Table 7.4   Status after 2 years of 700 consecutive patients discharged from a men's medical ward*

Status	% of patients
Well	27
Little change	15
Worse	10
Readmitted	23
Dead	25
Total	100

* After Ferguson and McPhail.

that only 27% of patients were well 2 years after discharge reflects the heavy preponderance of chronic and incurable conditions.

A natural response to this is to study the development of these illnesses before they become clinically apparent, in the hope of identifying treatable antecedents. A useful model of a chronic disease is to divide its evolution into three phases. In the precursor phase, abnormalities (for example an elevated serum cholesterol) are present without recognizable disease. In the preclinical phase, the disease is established but asymptomatic. In the clinical phase it is overt.

In clinical practice chronic disease tends to present as a series of acute episodes that occur towards the end of a prolonged pathological process. Thus a diagnosis of chronic bronchitis is rarely made before middle age, yet studies of the earlier sickness absence records of such individuals have shown that from their first entry into employment they tend to have had more acute respiratory illnesses than their contemporaries. There is even evidence that the 'chesty' child may be the father of the bronchitic man, suggesting a time span for the disease of 40 years or more.

In western populations atherosclerosis begins in childhood, and in young adults the coronary arteries are often already severely affected; yet clinical disease is rare before the age of about 35 years, by which time prevention or treatment are incompletely effective. In osteoarthritis symptoms are a late and relatively infrequent complication of many years of radiologically apparent changes. Adult hypertension may originate in infancy. These examples illustrate how the pathologically critical stages of chronic disease often occur long before the patient comes to medical care. Therefore these stages can be identified only by population studies.

In clinical practice cancers often appear to have an abrupt onset followed by rapid progression. The accessibility of the uterine cervix to exfoliative cytology first showed that dysplasia and in situ malignancy might antedate invasive disease by many years. Painstaking routine microscopy of apparently normal autopsy material has since shown that this is often found with other cancers too (see Table 6.1). Clinical cases of invasive disease may be only the extreme tail of a whole distribution of pathology, the rare complication of the common condition of in situ malignancy, which in turn may be an infrequent sequel of other kinds of dysplasia.

Identification of preclinical disease is the basis of screening, which is discussed in the next chapter. Among studies of the precursor phase, the Framingham study is one of the best known. Some 5000 people aged from 30 to 59 years have been examined annually over a 30-year period, and initial levels of serum lipids and other measurements correlated with subsequent morbidity and mortality. There have since been many similar studies. A recent one in Britain included serial measurements of the forced expiratory volume (FEV_1) in 800 men over an 8-year period. The lack of correlation between sputum production and the rate of decline of FEV_1 led to the concept of chronic bronchitis as two disorders which frequently coincide but are not usually related. Studies such as these are an essential part of our attempts to arrest and prevent chronic disease.

8. Screening

Screening in clinical practice

Modern hospital medicine is largely concerned with the care of patients who are in the later stages of chronic and incurable diseases such as atherosclerosis, malignancy, and mental illness. In these circumstances it is natural that doctors should seek to counteract the diseases by earlier diagnosis and treatment before irreparable damage has occurred. The development of techniques for mass examination has now made earlier diagnosis a practical possibility. At the same time population studies have revealed the large reservoir in the community of undiagnosed chronic disease. Out of these developments has arisen the current keen interest in screening.

Recent discussions of screening have tended to centre around the question of creating large national services. It is often forgotten that informal screening is basic to normal clinical practice. History-taking and physical examination of patients include a routine search for many conditions other than those that are suspected in the particular case. Blood pressure is measured, the mucosae inspected, the breasts palpated, and the urine tested. These all constitute screening (that is, the routine search for unsuspected disease), and this screening for hypertension, anaemia, breast cancer, diabetes, chronic renal disease and many other disorders is, rightly or wrongly, part of normal clinical practice.

Mass screening surveys

Mass screening surveys form one of the meeting points between epidemiology and clinical practice. The methods appropriate to mass examinations are epidemiological, but the objective is clinical action for individuals. Although both disciplines are involved, each needs to face some basic differences from its more usual area of practice.

Morbidity survey methods are designed primarily to characterize populations. For example, in estimating the community prevalence of depression it does not much matter if some individuals are misclassified, provided that the total count is about right. In screening, the priorities are reversed. The total count is not so important, but misclassification of individuals can lead to serious errors of management: treatment may be withheld from those who need it or given to others who do not.

In clinical practice it is the patient who takes the initiative in asking the doctor for help, but in screening it is the medical team which seeks out people who are symptom-free and tells some of them that their health is endangered. Epidemiological surveys have repeatedly shown that there is much undiagnosed disease in the community. For example, cross-sectional surveys have shown that something like 10% of middle-aged men have changes suggestive of ischaemia in their resting electrocardiograms, and the proportion is even higher if post-exercise records are available. From longitudinal studies it is clear that in comparison with their contemporaries these men are at a higher risk of death from coronary heart disease. Those whose medical experience has been exclusively in a clinical setting tend to think of diagnosis as something that is intrinsically worthwhile, an end in itself; as a result it is becoming fashionable to urge people to have a periodic 'health check-up' including electrocardiography. Before such a practice becomes widespread it is well to recall that, although a substantial minority will suffer major illness or death, more than 80% will still be alive and in normal health 5 years later. Furthermore, to tell someone that their heart is not normal may cause them serious anxiety, and currently there is no evidence that treatment is effective in such cases. Only when such treatment becomes available will there be adequate grounds for seeking to diagnose latent myocardial ischaemia.

Screening cannot be justified simply because it leads to more diagnoses. In the course of achieving these new diagnoses some costs are inevitably incurred as a result of that effort involved and the alarm caused to persons who previously believed themselves to be fit. These costs must be offset by evidence of commensurate benefit. More specifically, one needs to know the extent to which prognosis can be improved as a result of earlier diagnosis. This requires not only that there shall be an effective treatment, but that earlier treatment is more effective than later treatment.

Critical assessment of the benefits of screening poses a number of questions.

What is 'a case'?

The problems of case definition were discussed in Chapter 3 where it was seen that the more or less clear division between cases and normals in clinical practice is an artefact of the selection process leading to medical consultation. In the population disease exists in all grades of severity, and mild forms often greatly outnumber severe forms. Screening for glucose intolerance, for example, may identify as many as 10 'borderliners' for every one new case of frank diabetes. The variables by which a diseased state is recognized commonly follow a continuous, unimodal distribution, and this makes it difficult to define screening criteria for 'a case'.

The problem with regard to hypertension is illustrated by considering the population distribution of blood pressure. Somewhere towards the upper end of the distribution there is a level where treatment is necessary in order to reduce the risk of stroke, heart failure and renal damage. This level defines the cases that screening aims to discover and it is determined from all available evidence, particularly that from controlled trials. It will vary according to age, sex and other factors, and it will change as new treatments are introduced and new trials are reported. There may be disagreement on the precise level, but every doctor who measures the blood pressure of symptomless individuals should have defined criteria for therapy.

Although screening is undertaken simply in order to identify those individuals whose results exceed the critical level for intervention, inevitably it will also uncover large numbers of borderline cases. For blood pressure measurement these are people whose pressures fall below the treatment level but are still elevated to a degree that implies an impaired prognosis. They cannot truthfully be told that the results of screening are normal, but if they receive a less reassuring report and are not treated then screening may have done them a disservice.

What is the natural history of the condition?

The benefits of screening can be assessed only with reference to the outcome without it. Clinical experience of prognosis is of little assistance since clinical cases differ from the more numerous but milder cases detected by screening. There is the further problem (see p. 36) that the diagnostic implications of a clinical finding often vary according to the context in which it is observed. When plasma electrolyte levels are measured in hospital patients with hypertension, then hypokalaemia can be attributed to either diuretic therapy or possibly hyperaldosteronism; but when the same finding is uncovered by mass biochemical screening it is more likely to be due to an extreme of normal physiological variation.

Despite the fact that clinical experience may be a poor guide to the prognosis of screening findings, it may nevertheless inhibit further enquiry. Since it is known that intra-epithelial carcinoma of the cervix sometimes progresses to invasive disease it has proved difficult to set up a study to discover how often this occurs. Without knowledge of the natural history of the condition, the case for screening cannot be weighed.

Does earlier treatment improve the prognosis?

It may be easy to establish that certain individuals are at special risk of a disease but difficult to show that this risk can be reduced as a result of screening. For example, persons with clinically inapparent diabetes certainly have an increased mortality, but two randomized controlled trials have failed to show that the prognosis is improved by treatment. In the trial in Bedford, England, mortality after 10 years was similar in a group treated by tolbutamide and in the control group; and in an American trial cardiovascular mortality was reported as higher in patients who received either tolbutamide or phenformin than in controls. This indicates that there are currently no grounds for screening for symptomless cases.

The situation with regard to the early detection for lung cancer is similarly disappointing. By the time the disease is clinically diagnosed fewer than 25% of cases are resectable. However, there is evidence that many cases which present clinically with a mass near the hilum have originated in a peripheral and thus more operable situation. Such lesions may be detectable radiologically, the yield in surveys of middle-aged men being of the order of 1 per 1000 at the first examination. If not detected by screening it would be expected that most of these cases would have become inoperable by the time of normal clinical diagnosis. Here the

Table 8.1 Results of a randomized controlled trial of X-ray screening for lung cancer*

	No. of patients	
	6-monthly X-ray	Initial and final X-ray only
No. detected by X-ray	65	17
Resectable	42 (65%)	11 (65%)
Lung cancer deaths/1000/year	0.70	0.79

* Brett G Z 1968 Thorax 23: 414

possibility of benefit to a few people must be set against the discomfort and risks of surgery to a much larger number.

In such circumstances only a controlled trial can resolve the uncertainty. A group of 50 000 men participating in a mass X-ray service were divided randomly into 2 groups. For 3 years 1 group was X-rayed 6-monthly, but the other group was X-rayed only at the start and end of the period. Table 8.1 summarizes the findings. Screening evidently increased the detection rate and the number of operations; unfortunately the difference in lung cancer mortality was too small to be either statistically significant or practically important.

In other instances the improvement of prognosis by early detection has been clearly established. Rhesus haemolytic disease of the newborn is now a preventable disease, since 'at risk' mothers can be detected by screening and their subsequent sensitization by fetal red cells can be prevented by post-partum administration of anti-D antiserum. Screening for phenylketonuria in the neonatal period permits affected infants to be given a diet low in phenylalanine before the onset of irreversible mental changes (although trials are needed to discover how long this diet needs to be continued). Screening for symptomless hypertension in middle-aged men has been shown to yield a rewarding number of cases where timely treatment can much reduce the risk of stroke. In other instances, such as anaemia and glaucoma, theoretical hopes for screening have not been substantiated.

Assessment of screening test

The principles of assessment of screening tests are the same as for tests used in epidemiological surveys (pp. 32–37), the two basic components being *repeatability* and *validity*.

Repeatability

Repeatability influences the extent to which a single screening measurement may be taken as a sufficient guide to action. Where within-subject variability is large, as in blood pressure levels, repeated measurements are taken on separate occasions and averaged. Where observer variation is large, as in reading chest X-ray films for early tuberculosis, accuracy is improved by independent replicate readings. Where the result is much influenced by the particular technique or by the conditions under which it is made, this must be considered when determining the critical level above which action is initiated; the critical level of blood pressure, for example, should be higher for a hospital doctor than for a general practitioner's nurse-receptionist.

Validity

A screening test should be cheap, simple and quick, and so it is commonly not the best diagnostic measure of a disease. Its validity may be assessed by comparing it with the results of a reference test, usually full clinical investigation. Two kinds of error may be revealed, namely false positive and false negative classifications. False positive results lead to needless alarms and wasted investigations, whereas false negative results may lead to some people not receiving treatment from which they would benefit. A *specific* test is one that yields few false positives. These two components of validity are calculated by first setting up a '2 × 2' contingency table, as shown in Table 8.2. A worked example of this table is given in Table 3.2 (p. 37).

The proportion of true positives correctly identified $a/(a + c)$ is known as the *sensitivity* of the test. A high sensitivity is important when false negative errors are serious as, for example, when screening for chorionic carcinoma by measurement of gonado-trophins in women with a history of hydatidiform mole.

The proportion of true negatives correctly identified $d/(b + d)$ is known as the *specificity* of the test. Specific tests are necessary when false positive errors are undesirable either in terms of anxiety and discomfort to the subjects, or because they lead to further expensive investigations. Unfortunately attempts to make a test more specific, by raising the threshold for a positive case, usually have

Table 8.2 A contingency table relating the results of screening and reference tests

	Reference test		
	Positive	Negative	
Screening test			
Positive	True positives correctly identified (a)	False positives (b)	*Total positives by screening* (a + b)
Negative	False negatives (c)	True negatives correctly identified (d)	*Total negatives by screening* (c + d)
	Total true positives (a + c)	*Total true negatives* (b + d)	*Grand total* (a + b + c + d)

the effect of making it less sensitive. The appropriate balance is a matter for judgement in any particular situation.

When a test is first applied in a new situation it is not sufficient to know only the levels of sensitivity and specificity. One needs to know in addition the likelihood that a person with a positive test has the disease, i.e. the *predictive value* of a positive test, and conversely, the likelihood that a person with a negative test has not got the disease. Using the scheme in Table 8.2 the predictive value of a positive test is calculated as $a/(a + b)$, and that of a negative test as $d/(c + d)$. It is important to note that predictive values, and hence also the performance of the test, depend on the prevalence of disease in the particular group. A value for specificity may seem sufficient and yet when prevalence is low the false positives may be unexpectedly numerous. Figure 8.1 shows the performance of a test with a 95% specificity and sensitivity. As the prevalence of the disease increases from 0 to 100% so does the predictive value of a positive test.

Understanding this point is of practical importance. New diagnostic tests are usually tried first in hospitals or clinics, where the prevalence of disease is high; but a decision to use them for population screening requires data on their performance in low prevalence situations. An ELISA test for human immuno-deficiency virus (HIV) antibodies is highly sensitive (99%) and specific (97%), and when it is used in suspected clinical cases most of the results will be true; but when applied to screening of blood donors, if the prevalence of true positives is 1:10 000 the false positive results will outnumber true verdicts by 300 to 1.

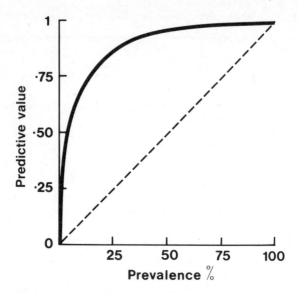

Fig. 8.1   Relationship between disease prevalence and the predictive value of a positive result of a screening test with 95% sensitivity and specificity.

Evaluation of a screening service

The ideal screening programme is one in which a cheap and safe test identifies a large group of people in whom prognosis is bad and treatment is effective. For example, among babies born alive with a birth-weight less than 2000 g there occur around half of all neonatal deaths. This, with the information that facilities for special care can reduce neonatal mortality, establishes the great importance of identifying this high-risk group. Unfortunately in most other instances the costs of screening tests are much greater, the yield is smaller, and the benefits less certain.

Costs of the test

These need to be measured both as they affect the patients, in terms of time lost, discomfort and anxiety, and as they affect the resources of the health services. For breast cancer screening it was found that identification of one new case required the examination by palpation and mammography of 170 women and the taking of nine biopsies.

Yield

The summarizing figure for yield is the number of tests that must be done in order to identify one case whose prognosis will be improved as a result of early detection. Many conditions for which screening might be considered have too low a prevalence to justify routine examination of the whole population. Among inborn metabolic errors, for example, phenylketonuria has a prevalence of about 1 in 10 000, and this is considered to justify routine screening. Wilson's disease equally calls for early recognition and treatment, but unfortunately with a prevalence less than 1 in 100 000 the yield may be unacceptably low.

Sometimes it may be possible to improve the yield by restricting screening to some readily identifiable high-risk group. For example the incidence of chorionic carcinoma following normal pregnancy is 1 per 50 000, too low a yield to justify screening. Following hydatidiform mole the incidence is about 25%, so that screening is clearly justified despite the cost of the test.

Policy decisions

From a recent Swedish trial the balance sheet in Table 8.3 can be derived. For every woman who was alive at the end of the trial as a result of screening (an average up to that point of an extra 2.5 years of life), 1850 had to be screened. About 75 women were submitted to the anxiety and trouble of investigating a false positive report, and in a further 15 the positive test result was correct but the outcome was not altered: the women were simply made aware of the diagnosis earlier. On the other hand, about 1800 women received the benefit of reassurance from a negative report. These results show once again that policy decisions require judgements. They do not follow automatically from the data, but yet the data are necessary.

Table 8.3   The balance sheet for breast cancer screening

Gains	Losses
1 extra survivor (2.5+ years)	Costs to medical services and women of screening 1850 women
1800 reassured	*c.* 75 false positive reports; 15 correctly identified, without benefit

The final decision to initiate a screening service depends on the balancing of many factors to yield an overall estimate of the cost, to the patient and the health service, of preventing one pathological event. This balance is made difficult by the different kinds of unit in which each factor is measured: there is no scientific basis for determining exchange rates between discomfort, survival and money.

9. Epidemics

Epidemics of infectious diseases, such as plague, cholera, typhus and typhoid, have profoundly influenced European history, and remain an important threat to many tropical countries. Modern epidemiology arose out of the study of such classical epidemics, explosive outbreaks of disease affecting many people and due to infections or in some instances to dietary deficiency or poisoning. In 1854 Dr John Snow showed that the outbreak of cholera around Broad Street in London resulted from contamination of drinking water with excrement from cholera sufferers. This brilliant discovery, made 30 years before the description of the cholera vibrio, was a remarkable justification of a simple and well-conceived epidemiological study.

Infectious disease epidemics

In Europe and North America epidemics of infectious disease remain common, although their extent and severity is less than in previous times. Influenza remains an important cause of death, especially among the elderly and chronic sick. In the 1957–58 influenza epidemic the death rate in England and Wales was 1 per 1000 population above the seasonal average. An estimated 12 million people developed the disease and there was a 5-fold rise in the volume of general practitioners' work.

In the summer of 1981 the first recognized cases of acquired immune deficiency syndrome (AIDS) occurred in America. *Pneumocystis carinii* pneumonia and Kaposi's sarcoma were reported in young men, who were subsequently found to be both homosexual and immunocompromised. Figure 9.1 shows the alarming early rise in the numbers of cases in the United Kingdom, and the later continuing rise but lengthening of the doubling time.

More mundanely, outbreaks of diseases such as mumps, measles,

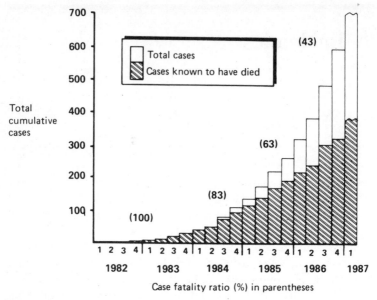

Fig. 9.1   Number of cases of acquired immunodeficiency syndrome in the UK.

rubella, streptococcal infection and food poisoning remain commonplace; and outbreaks of rarer diseases such as hepatitis B and typhoid occur from time to time. Although medical officers in charge of institutions, hospitals, schools, barracks and factories are more liable than others to be confronted by infectious disease epidemics, any doctor may be called upon at short notice to assist in the management of one.

In some epidemics the challenge is one of diagnosis. Diseases such as brucellosis and legionnaire's disease are not always readily diagnosed clinically, and the clinical manifestations associated with a particular infectious agent may vary from one time to another.

A general distinction is made between point-source and contagious disease epidemics. In a *point-source epidemic* many susceptible individuals are exposed, more or less simultaneously, to a source of pathogenic organisms, as when the guests at a wedding reception ate sausage meat contaminated with staphylococci. The result of such exposure is an explosive increase in the number of cases of disease over a short period. At the wedding the vomiting caused by the staphylococcal toxin began in a few hours. In contrast, organisms in a *contagious disease epidemic* are propagated in the community by passage from person to person,

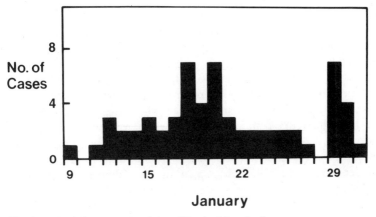

Fig. 9.2 An influenza outbreak in a Wensleydale school.

so that the initial rise in the number of cases is less abrupt than in point-source epidemics.

Figure 9.2 shows an outbreak of influenza in Wensleydale, one of several epidemics described in Pickles' classic book *Epidemiology in A Country Practice:*

> . . . a particularly worthy schoolmistress returned to her home after a Christmas holiday spent with her relatives. On the morning of the school opening, knowing that she was ill, with commendable if mistaken zeal, she attended her school. In the afternoon she was utterly unable to return, but from that brief morning session a crop of 78 cases resulted.

The slow rise in daily numbers of cases after 9 January when the schoolmistress fell ill is characteristic of contagious disease epidemics.

A feature of non-industrialized countries is the multiplicity of *endemic* infectious diseases, which form the dominant health problem. The term endemic implies the habitual presence of a disease or agent of disease within a given area. Many endemic diseases rapidly become epidemic if environmental or host influences change in a way that favours transmission. Ecological changes may favour breeding of an insect vector; non-immune persons may accumulate in a population as a result of births or immigration from non-endemic areas; or the epidemic may be heralded by an *epizootic* (an epidemic among animals) such as occurs among rats before an outbreak of human plague.

Epidemics of non-infectious disease

While industrialization has led to a decline in infectious disease, it has brought new forms of epidemic. A number of large-scale epidemics have arisen from chemical contaminants. Outbreaks of organic mercury poisoning, with resulting deaths and neurological disability, have been reported from Iraq, Pakistan and Guatemala as a result of ingestion of wheat treated with methyl- and ethylmercury compounds. This wheat was intended only for use as seed, and warnings that it had been treated with mercury to prevent fungus infection and was, therefore, unfit to eat, were not understood by farmers. In Spain in 1981 20 000 people were affected by a new disease, named the 'toxic allergic syndrome', the most striking feature of which was a pneumonopathy. During the first four months of the epidemic more than 100 people died and 13 000 were treated in hospital. Investigation showed that the cause was ingestion of olive oil adulterated with rapeseed oil. The oil contained aniline (a colourant used to denature rapeseed oil for industrial use) and chemical products of an attempt to refine out the aniline.

Widespread environmental contamination is a new agent of epidemic disease. In the United States in 1973 a fire retardant chemical, polybrominated biphenyl, was inadvertently mixed with farm feed. The contaminated meat and dairy products that resulted led to most of Michigan's 9 million citizens having detectable levels of the chemical in their blood. The effects on their health are not known.

Recently in Britain an increased incidence of luekaemia has been found among children born in the vicinity of the Sellafield nuclear waste reprocessing plant. The discovery of high concentrations of aluminium in senile plaque, the specific pathological feature of the brains of patients with Alzheimer's disease, has implicated aluminium as a possible cause of the disease. Suspicion has increased with the discovery that differences in disease rates in the country correlate with differing aluminium concentrations in drinking water.

The explosion at the Chernobyl nuclear power station on 26 April 1986 illustrates a new form of point-source epidemic. Two workers at the plant died almost immediately and a further 29 died within the next month or so. Large amounts of radioactive material were released into the environment and were spread throughout Europe.

In current usage, the term epidemic is applied to any pronounced

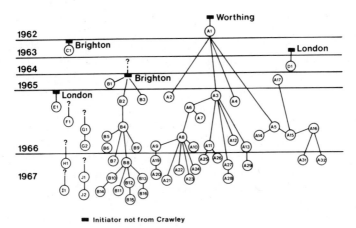

■ Initiator not from Crawley

Fig. 9.3 The spread of heroin abuse among 58 young people living in Crawley in 1967. (Source: Alarcon R de 1969 WHO Bulletin of narcotics 21: 17)

rise in incidence or prevalence rates and is not restricted to explosive outbreaks. The time period is no longer confined to a few weeks or months. The increases in coronary heart disease, lung cancer, traffic accidents and self-poisoning during the past few decades are examples of modern slow epidemics of non-communicable disease.

Figure 9.3 shows another form of epidemic, related to abuse of drugs. Among young people in Crawley the spread of heroin abuse mimicked transmission of a contagious disease.

Not only the abuse of medication but also its side-effects seem likely to be a continuing source of epidemics. Clinicians have a special responsibility in the early detection of iatrogenic epidemics, such as that of phocomelia due to thalidomide, or of deaths in asthmatics due to pressurized bronchodilator aerosols, or of corneal damage, skin rashes and a variety of other adverse effects of practolol.

Investigation of epidemics

Since epidemic diseases occur widely among animals and plants much can be learnt about their investigation and control from biologists in many fields. Veterinary surgeons encounter a variety of epidemics, including infectious disease epidemics (e.g. foot and mouth disease of cattle), deficiency disease epidemics (e.g. sway-back of lambs, associated with copper deficiency) and epidemics due to chemicals (such as occurred recently with arsenic-contaminated calf feed). Zoologists have made detailed studies of control methods for epidemics of locusts and other insects. Plant epidemiologists have developed techniques whereby epidemics of important plant diseases such as potato blight may be predicted using meteorological and other data. In these fields sophisticated technique such as computer simulation have been applied to the study of epidemics, and these likewise find an application in the study of human epidemics.

It is, however, the purpose of this chapter merely to describe the practical steps that should be taken by clinicians during the management of limited epidemics. Management of large-scale epidemics, like that of large-scale disasters, requires the services of many people and is outside the responsibilities of the individual doctor. AIDS, though now a large-scale epidemic, provides a good example of the practical management of an epidemic.

In the investigation of epidemics it is wise to follow a systematic routine, even though public reaction, urgency and the local situation may make this difficult. The steps listed below need not always be undertaken in the order given and some will be done concurrently.

Verification of diagnosis

At the outset of any investigation it is necessary that the diagnosis made on the cases should be verified. A doctor called to an outbreak of 'food poisoning' is unwise to begin by collecting information about recent meals before confirming that the clinical history of the patients is compatible with the diagnosis. With some diseases, such as Lassa fever, the urgency of the situation demands that immediate action is taken on the basis of a clinical diagnosis alone, although laboratory confirmation can be obtained subsequently. For most diseases there is less urgency and there is time to confirm the diagnosis before any further steps are taken. Three patients with halothane-induced hepatitis were recently referred to a university hospital over a short period. Investigation of an outbreak of infectious hepatitis was begun, presumably because the clustering of cases gave an impression of infectivity and unduly influenced the physician's diagnosis.

From time to time, errors in collecting, handling or processing laboratory specimens may cause 'pseudo-epidemics'. The Center for Disease Control in Atlanta has reported a number of such pseudo-epidemics. For example, an apparent outbreak of typhoid occurred when specimen contamination produced blood cultures positive for *Salmonella typhi* in six patients. Although such mishaps are rare, it is the clinician's role to ensure that laboratory findings correlate with the clinical state of the patients.

AIDS was originally defined by the occurrence of a disease which was at least moderately indicative of an underlying cellular immune deficiency, for example opportunistic infection or Kaposi's sarcoma in a patient aged less than 60 years, in a patient with no known cause for such immune deficiency. This initial definition was later modified because laboratory tests to detect antibody were developed, and because the clinical pattern of the disease changed.

Confirmation of the existence of an epidemic

If a disease is endemic it is necessary to estimate, at least approximately, its previous frequency before concluding that an epidemic exists. Pseudo-epidemics may be caused by a sudden increase in a doctor's awareness of a disease or by some change in the organisation of his or her practice which brings more cases to notice. Again from the Center for Disease Control comes the example of a pseudo-epidemic of staphylococcal diarrhoea in a nursery, which was reported after *Staphylococcus aureus* was isolated from two infants with loose stools. A subsequent review of medical records showed that there had been no real increase in the incidence of diarrhoeal disease in the nursery.

An epidemic has begun when the incidence of a disease rises above a normal endemic level. Various indices of endemicity may be used according to whether or not the disease has a cyclic pattern of occurrence. For diseases showing seasonal variations, the mean may be taken of incidence rates for particular weeks or months over the previous several years, or mean high and low levels over a period of years may be calculated.

A single case of botulism is considered as an outbreak needing investigation, but this is exceptional. Usually there must be at least two cases of a non-endemic disease occurring at one time and place to stimulate action. At an early stage of an epidemic a graph of the changing incidence of the disease should be drawn and the geographical distribution of the cases mapped.

The steep rise in the numbers of cases of AIDS, shown in Figure 9.1, rapidly established the existence of an epidemic. As it evolved, large geographical differences in rate became apparent. By 1987 there was almost 1 case per 1000 population in San Francisco and New York, where AIDS had become the commonest cause of death in young men. This was 7 times the rate in the USA as a whole.

Identification of cases and their characteristics

In order to build up a description of the epidemic it may be necessary to take a case history from each confirmed or suspected case. It is common to find that the cases that are notified or otherwise recorded are only a proportion of those with the disease, and additional cases must be sought. In some circumstances this search may depend on clinical examination to detect minor or modified forms of the disease. In other circumstances laboratory investigations may be needed, such as an Australian antigen test and liver function tests in convalescent patients suspected of having had hepatitis B. The history taken will include basic details of the patient and his or her illness (e.g. time of onset of symptoms, recent movements), and more detailed questioning on matters relevant to the particular disease (e.g. meals eaten, if food poisoning is suspected). From these case histories will come a profile of those with the disease from which, by relating the profile to data on the entire population at risk, it will be possible to calculate incidence rates for age, sex and other subgroups. In addition the case histories may identify an experience that is common to those affected by the disease but not shared by those seemingly exposed but not affected.

In epidemics of serious contagious disorders identification of cases is followed by listing of possible source contacts whom the patients encountered around the presumed time of infection and of contacts whom the patient could subsequently have infected. These contacts are then interviewed and investigated as necessary.

Because of the variety of its clinical presentations some cases of AIDS may go unrecorded. This is especially likely to have happened in the early years of the epidemic, before the discovery of the human immunodeficiency virus (HIV) in 1983 and the development of an antibody test in 1984. The extent of local outbreaks may have been underestimated. Case histories focus on homosexual practices, intravenous drug abuse, blood transfusions and high-risk heterosexual partners as the main sources of infection.

Definition and investigation of the population at risk

For a number of reasons investigation of an epidemic may necessitate close study of the population at risk, or a sample of it, in addition to study of the cases themselves. In the investigation of subacute myelo-optic neuropathy (SMON), a neurological disease which recently appeared in Japan, one of the pieces of evidence linking the disease with the antidiarrhoeal drug clioquinol was the observation that in hospitals and clinics where the disease was not seen the drug was not in use.

Definition of the population at risk enables the extent and severity of an epidemic to be expressed in terms of rates, such as the following. The *attack rate* relates the number of cases to the total population at risk, and may be either *crude* or *age/sex-specific*. The *secondary attack rate* in a contagious disease epidemic is based on the number of cases occurring after introduction of the primary case, this number being then related either to the total population at risk or the susceptible population only (that is, those who are not immune). The *case fatality ratio* relates the number of deaths to the number of cases, either clinical cases alone or both clinical and subclinical ones.

The antibody test for HIV infection has given a clearer understanding of how the epidemic evolved. Tests on stored samples of serum collected from homosexual men in San Francisco showed that 4% of samples taken in 1978 were HIV positive. For blood taken in 1980 the figure was 24%. These, and similar observations elsewhere, suggest that the proportion of individuals affected needs to be high before cases of AIDS appear. A more recent increase in the prevalence of HIV infection has been seen in other groups, for example 6% in 1980 to 76% in 1985 among intravenous drug users in southern Italy. Among drug users in Italy who are also prostitutes the prevalence is 70%.

Formulation of a hypothesis as to the source and spread of the epidemic

Investigation of cases and the population at risk, and consideration of relevant environmental changes, may enable formulation of a hypothesis on the origin of the epidemic. Sometimes confirmation of this hypothesis has to await the results of special investigations, such as analysis of water supplies or identification of insect vectors. At other times action to control the epidemic must be taken before investigations are complete. On the basis of suggestive but incomplete evidence a decision was taken to ban clioquinol in Japan. The decline in frequency of SMON is one of the observations made subsequently that has strengthened the evidence that the drug was causative.

The ideal outcome of an investigation is a complete picture of the critical changes that led to the epidemic, of the source, transmission and mode of entry of the disease agent, of its characteristics, and of the varying susceptibility of individuals in the population. This ideal is often not realized.

Both in the USA and in Britain the first wave of the AIDS epidemic occurred in homosexual men, and the next and current wave is among intravenous drug abusers. HIV has been isolated from many body fluids, among which semen, blood and possibly cervical secretions are especially infectious. The commonest method of its transmission is homosexual intercourse. Other methods are through contaminated needles, transfusion with infected blood or blood products, receipt of donated organs or semen, and from mother to child in utero. The next wave of the epidemic may occur in the heterosexual population. Case reports and epidemiological studies clearly show that the virus can be transmitted from men to women and from women to men. In Africa HIV is mainly spread by heterosexual intercourse.

Management of epidemics

Management of an epidemic in a community is analogous to managing acute illnesses in clinical practice. On the one hand timely action can save life, on the other, many patients recover unaided and misplaced intervention can do harm. It is the nature of epidemic disease to wax and wane in frequency. An epidemic will die down either when the number of susceptible people is sufficiently reduced (by acquisition of immunity, by death, or by migration), or when environmental conditions become unfavourable to the disease agent, for example by exhaustion of the source or a change in climate. However, the reasons for the decline of a particular epidemic often remain a matter of speculation. We do not know why plague disappeared from England in 1666, nor why the incidence of leprosy fluctuates in different parts of the world. Against a background of fluctuating disease incidence doctors may readily get credit for ineffective control measures which happen to coincide with a downward trend.

Treatment of cases

The treatment of numerous cases during an epidemic may pose problems of accommodation, staffing and the availability of medical supplies. To meet the demand for hospital beds during an influenza epidemic it may be necessary to discontinue non-emergency procedures. In countries with well-developed medical services demands for additional staffing can usually be met, but in non-industrialized countries an epidemic of cholera may require rapid training of auxiliaries, students, service personnel or any available manpower. Needs for drugs and equipment must be forecast, and the timely organization of physiotherapy and rehabilitation may reduce the aftermath of disability. As they have grown up it has been possible to anticipate the needs of children affected by thalidomide many years in advance.

AIDS is a costly disease, because of its often prolonged course and the variety of its complications. The estimated lifetime hospital cost of looking after a patient in Britain is £7000–20 000. The number of patients, however, was only around 1000 by 1987.

Control measures

In contagious disease epidemics, affected individuals may require isolation, and quarantine may have to be imposed to prevent movement in or out of the area. It may be necessary to locate contacts and keep them under surveillance. Other epidemics may necessitate immediate cessation of sales of food, the withdrawal of a drug, or closure of a ward or institution. Whatever the urgency for commencing control measures, time must also be found to explain the situation to the community at risk and to ensure their co-operation. Public co-operation is often critical in epidemic control.

After immediate control measures have been put into effect more permanent changes such as improvements in hygiene or alteration in industrial practices can be initiated.

The major strategy for control of AIDS is health information, aimed at changing behaviour. Those at risk of sexual transmission are counselled to adopt safer sexual practices, have fewer partners, know about their partners' sexual and drug history, and use a condom. Other advice is directed at preventing transmission in those who inject drugs, transmission by blood, blood products and organ donation, and vertical transmission.

Surveillance

After an epidemic is under control it may be necessary to keep the community under surveillance to detect further rises in incidence and ensure the effectiveness of control measures. At a local level surveillance will depend upon clinical records, data from sources such as public health laboratories and veterinary services, or observations by special surveillance staff such as the hospital cross-infection officer. At a national level data come from the routine sources described in Chapter 2.

In many countries schemes for notification of infectious and occupational diseases and of congenital malformations have been set up to facilitate early detection and control of epidemics. The increasing recognition of environmental hazards, due to substances introduced by humans into the environment as a result of the application of new technology, has led to a demand for large-scale surveillance systems based on automated record linkage. Whether or not such systems come into operation, clinicians' awareness of changes in disease frequency or of the appearance of clusters of unusual cases will continue to be crucial to the early detection of epidemics.

10. Epidemiology in the planning and evaluation of medical services

Medical services are expensive and no country in the world has resources of trained staff, equipment and buildings sufficient to meet the population's need for health care. There seems to be no limit to the resources that could be expended on improving health, and it follows that the needs of one group of people, say expectant mothers, must be weighed against those of other groups, say geriatric patients or chronic schizophrenics. Although resources could be allocated to one or other group purely on the basis of a subjective judgement (and in many countries the chronic mentally sick are traditionally given lowest priority), the ideal of a health service that is equally available to the whole population requires that the benefits yielded by resources allocated to one group of people should be measured objectively, and compared with similar measurements when resources are allocated to other groups.

Evaluation of health services is necessary not only for allocation of resources at national, regional or district level but also to ensure that the health services adapt to changing demands upon them, consequent upon changing patterns of disease, the introduction of new therapies, or changes in public attitudes. Furthermore, the scarcity of resources lays an obligation on each doctor to utilize the money and manpower at his or her disposal with maximum effectiveness. This obligation requires doctors to monitor their clinical policies by measurement of immediate and long-term consequences, and to attempt to allocate their time and the facilities at their disposal in a way that is appropriate to the needs of all patients, and not only to those who demand care most pressingly by reason of life-threatening or potentially curable illness.

Thus evaluation should be a normal activity of all doctors. This requires an understanding of epidemiological principles. Neither a regional renal dialysis programme nor the treatment of hyper-

Table 10.1 Variation between different areas of the USA in the percentage of people who have had organs removed surgically

Organ	Age (years)	% of persons	
		Low area	High area
Tonsils	20	6	68
Uterus	70	20	75
Prostate	80	20	80

tension within a general practice can be evaluated without knowledge of epidemiological techniques such as the measurement of morbidity and survival rates. The role of epidemiology in evaluation is two-fold. Firstly, since groups of patients are studied, techniques of measurement applicable to groups are required. Secondly, epidemiology serves to relate findings made on groups to the whole population. The need to consider health services within the context of the whole population is illustrated by Table 10.1, which shows the astonishing differences in the frequency of tonsillectomy, hysterectomy and prostatectomy in different areas of the USA. Clearly these figures do not reflect only differences in the frequency of diseases for which removal of the organs was considered to be beneficial, but resulted from other influences, such as differing opinions on the indications for surgery. Such data, of which there are many other examples, demand that further investigation is carried out into the actual need for surgery and the extent to which this need is being met or more than met.

Epidemiology is only one of a number of disciplines, ranging from pharmacology to sociology, which must be brought to bear in evaluation. Its role has, however, been reinforced by the number of epidemiologists who have recently taken an interest in this field. Concern with the distribution of disease, and the pioneer use of controlled trials to evaluate preventive measures such as vaccines, has led epidemiologists to study the methodological problems of evaluation.

Need, demand, outcome and planning

If the achievements of health services are to be quantified it is necessary to define measurable outcomes of the treatment and care they provide. It is self-evident that achievement can be measured only if objectives are first agreed upon and then a measure made of the extent to which they have been fulfilled. For disorders such as strangulated hernia or bacterial meningitis the primary outcome may be defined simply as survival or death. In these circumstances it is possible to use as an index the case fatality rate, which is available from routine data.

Usually the outcome of treatment cannot be adequately described in terms of survival and it is necessary to measure grades of disability, or the extent of lesions or, most complex of all, the quality of life. The justification of arterial surgery to correct atherosclerotic occlusion in the leg must come from measurement of the patients' ability subsequently to work, be socially independent, or in some way lead a 'better' life than previously. If the measures of outcome are inadequate the value of therapy may be concealed. One of the contributions of social science to medicine will be the development of techniques that will assess comfort and other feelings which make up the quality of life. The evaluation of many aspects of psychiatric treatment must be attendant on these developments, and there is an especial need for them in services, such as those for the mentally subnormal, where the principle objective is to care for the patients rather than alter the natural history of a pathological process. Although the quantification of outcome is an important step towards an objective assessment of medical services, the final comparison of different kinds of outcome must remain subjective. Surgical treatment of osteosarcoma of the leg may sometimes improve the outcome in terms of long-term survival but worsen it in terms of the quality of life during the survival period. The choice between longer survival or greater well-being is a matter of personal preference.

An important aspect of the effectiveness of a service is the extent to which it matches the demands and needs of the population. *Demand* for a service may arise from patients or doctors. Patients perceive that they *need* a service, and hence demand it, although the service may not be able to provide effective treatment for that need. Sometimes need may be unperceived by the patients, as in many psychiatric illnesses, and hence may not lead to demand. Doctors may initiate demand for a service, as has occurred for large-scale screening services. Demand in excess of actual need may originate from patients, doctors or from quite different sources, such as the pharmaceutical industry. The interrelationship of need and demand is shown diagrammatically in Figure 10.1

Need and demand for a service do not inevitably lead to

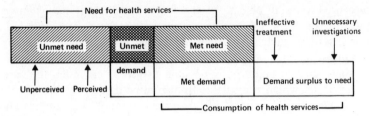

Fig. 10.1 The interrelationship of need and demand for health services.

utilization. Many people who need rehabilitation services, for example, do not utilize them because they do not know of their existence or how to gain access to them. Even when medical contact is established, this will not always result in sustained or effective treatment. This often occurs among patients with epilepsy, due to failure to take prescribed treatments or to the breakdown of follow-up arrangements. An aspect of effectiveness whose study is still in its infancy concerns the factors that determine patients' compliance with therapeutic regimens and with health education.

Our knowledge of the extent of unmet need in the community is fragmentary. In Britain the beginning of a systematic approach to measurement of need has been made by applying the techniques of the General Household Survey. Members of a sample of households are interviewed and asked for details of their illness and the care they have sought. Research surveys directed at specific problems have provided startling glimpses of the extent of unmet need. A survey of 200 elderly Scots revealed 38 with general medical problems which would have benefited from medical advice and 16 with depression. Remediable defects of vision and hearing were found, and impaired mobility due to untreated foot conditions was common.

There is good reason to think that in areas of medical care such as the diagnosis and treatment of deafness in the elderly, there is both a considerable unmet need, perceived and unperceived, and a considerable unmet demand due to the scarcity of resources for hearing tests and provision of hearing aids.

Cost

Clearly the limiting resources in a health service are not only financial but the time of skilled personnel. The effectiveness of advanced technical services such as cardiac surgery and renal

Table 10.2 Cost comparison of long-stay hospital and domiciliary care, 1972

	Annual cost (£)
Long-stay hospital	2970
Local authority home (+ nursing and medical services)	1410
Domiciliary care (+ nursing and medical services)	905–1995

Office of Health Economics 1979 Dementia in old age. OHE, London

dialysis has to be weighed against both their heavy financial costs and their utilization of the time of doctors, nurses, technicians and other staff who might otherwise be employed elsewhere in the health service. Sometimes it is necessary to consider the relative costs of providing alternative services to meet a particular need. Table 10.2 shows cost estimates for alternative forms of care for the elderly sick. Domiciliary care is cheapest, provided the patient lives with a family and no cost is included for family support; but it becomes more expensive than a local authority home if the patient lives alone in a house with high capital value or with a family, one of whose members is consequently unable to go out to work. Hospital care appears to be the most expensive, but this could reflect an inadequate assessment of help from other household members. The final balance should also take account of where the patient is happiest or lives longest, and these have not been measured.

The costing of medical care requires complex accountancy, but alternative indices related to use of resources have been used in evaluation studies. For example, different hospital discharge policies following herniorrhaphy have been 'costed' in terms of the number of days in hospital, the numbers of postoperative general practitioner consultations, and the duration of sickness absence from work. The burden of chronic disabilities such as rheumatoid arthritis may be crudely costed in terms of the social services used by patients.

Prescribing is an aspect of medical practice that is relatively easy to cost. Routinely, on about 1 month in 12, all prescriptions issued by general practitioners in Britain are sent to a central pricing unit. This identifies practitioners whose prescribing costs per patient are 25% above the average for the area. The prescribing pattern of each of these practitioners is then studied in detail and information fed back to them. This feedback is often followed by a marked reduction of prescribing costs.

Efficiency

The cost of therapeutic and preventive services in terms of manpower and money depend not only on the actual medical procedures carried out but on the way in which the services are organized. Among clinicians there is an increasing awareness of the need to optimize the use of personnel and materials and thereby increase efficiency. In general practice wide variations have been found in simple indices of workload such as the average number of consultations per list patient per year, or the relative frequency of consultations in the doctor's surgery as opposed to home visits. The variations revealed point to the need for studies of practice organization.

Length of stay in hospital for a number of common disorders varies remarkably from one hospital to another. In a recent study of inguinal herniorrhaphy the average stay in different hospitals within one region varied from 3.8 to 9.3 days. Such wide differences cannot be wholly rational (and indeed those consultants who worked in more than one hospital tended to conform to local custom rather than maintain a consistent policy). There would be a considerable increase in efficiency in the health service if the length of stay for such a common condition were shortened by even a few days — provided, of course, that the outcome was not jeopardized.

A randomized trial compared the outcome of uncomplicated acute myocardial infarction according to duration of bed-rest and hospitalization. One group of patients was mobilized after 1 week and discharged 2 weeks later; the other group was mobilized after 3 weeks and discharged 1 week after that. During the year following infarction, no difference was found between the groups either in mortality or in morbidity from recurrence of infarction, episodes of acute ischaemia, or congestive cardiac failure. The need for more controlled trials to measure the benefits of different lengths of stay for common illnesses is clear. Such trials have an important role in the evaluation of efficiency, but techniques of operational research and economics, outside the scope of doctors, may also be required.

Observational studies

The methods of evaluation studies are either observational or experimental. Observational studies are broadly of two kinds. Either groups of patients who have undergone treatment are followed up, or changes in the occurrence of a disease in the community are related to the usage of different therapies. Experimental studies, including randomized controlled trials, depend on the use of comparison groups exposed in the same planned way to different therapies.

The follow-up study was discussed in Chapter 7. Outside the framework of a formal follow-up a doctor's impressions of the long-term outcome of therapy tend to be biased. The dichotomy between hospital and domiciliary care makes it difficult for either hospital doctors or general practitioners to have a complete view of an illness. Perhaps hospital doctors, because of their brief association with most patients, are the especial victims of this. It is bizarre that the staff of coronary care units should sometimes have to read the announcements of deaths in local papers as the easiest way of discovering which of their patients have died after discharge. Undoubtedly far too few follow-up studies are carried out, and doctors seem to be needlessly inhibited from undertaking them by the belief that they necessarily require much time and expertise.

In general, observational data are sufficient only in the evaluation of treatments that are markedly effective. Figure 10.2 shows the sharp fall in maternal mortality attributable to sepsis, toxaemia and haemorrhage, which occurred from 1935 onwards. There is little doubt that much of this fall reflects improvements in obstetric care. Unfortunately most therapies do not effect such dramatic changes in health statistics and their evaluation requires an experimental study.

Experimental studies

The essence of the randomized controlled trial is that the outcome of a treatment given to one group of patients is compared with that in one or more other groups given different treatments or none at all. Allocation of individuals to the treatment and comparison groups is by random selection. Although randomization often evokes ethical objections from doctors, who properly wish to give the best treatment available to each patient coming under their care, there is no gainsaying the opposing viewpoint that without randomized trials the effectiveness of many treatments will never be measured. It is unethical to deny improvements in therapy to future patients because trials are not carried out.

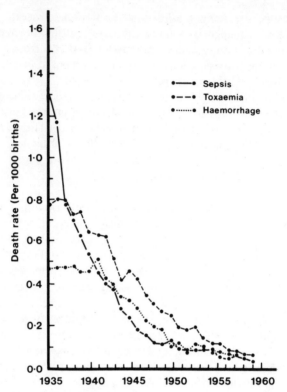

Fig. 10.2 Maternal mortality rates due to sepsis, toxaemia and haemorrhage in England and Wales. (Source: McKeown T, Lowe C R 1974 An introduction to social medicine. Blackwell, Oxford)

Random allocation of treatments in a trial avoids the biases that are introduced if the doctor allocates patients to one group or another by personal selection. Inevitably such selection tends to distribute patients with a less favourable prognosis unevenly, according to whether the doctor believes at the outset that the treatment being tried is better or worse than the alternative. There is also no doubt of the superiority of formal trials over clinical impressions in the detection of small differences in the effectiveness of therapies. The use of trials to test new drug regimens is well established, but it is unsatisfactory that major treatment policies should often become established without prior evaluation. Once therapies become established there can develop a consensus opinion that a trial is unethical. For this reason the benefits of coronary care units, for example, are still not clear.

Although the wider use of randomized trials, applied to policies of clinical management as well as to drugs, would lead to a more rational therapeutic approach, such trials are by no means perfect tools. Many trials include relatively small numbers of patients, and randomization may by chance lead to marked dissimilarities between treatment and comparison groups. Differences with respect to known variables such as age and sex may be allowed for during analysis, but patients may be heterogeneous in many ways of which the investigator is unaware.

Conclusion

Evaluation of treatment given will allow clinicians to maximize beneficial changes in the natural history of patients, to relate their activities to the actual needs of the population and not only to demands, and to minimize the resources used to meet a given need. In addition, doctors may have to justify the allocation of resources to their speciality before committees at district, regional or national level. The members of such committees can reasonably expect their medical advisers to present them with an objective and scientific summary of the benefits and disadvantages of any medical procedure being considered.

Appendix

Rates

Rates are used to express the numbers of people with a state (e.g. a pathological lesion) or the numbers of events (e.g. births or admissions to hospital) in relation to the total population at risk. All rates have a *time limit*, a *numerator* (measures of states or events) and a *denominator* (the population). Populations are groups of people, including both sick and healthy, defined by certain common characteristics, e.g. age, sex, residence, nationality or occupation. *Crude rates* are not standardized for age, sex or other variables. When it is necessary to take account of variations in the intensity or duration of exposure within a population, a denominator may be used other than the number of people in the related population. For example in the British Antarctic Survey the frequency of colds was given as 1.2 colds per 100 man-months spent in isolation compared with 25.2 colds per 100 man-months during the relief period when the supply ship called. Use of man-months as the denominator gave a rate that more accurately reflected the risk of a cold than one based on the total number of survey personnel. Similarly numbers of vehicle miles driven are often used as the denominator in rates expressing the frequency of road traffic accidents.

Birth rate. The number of births occurring per unit of population during a specified period of time. The crude (i.e. unstandardized) birth rate is usually calculated by relating total live births in a year to the total mid-year population. (Crude birth rate in England and Wales in 1985 was 13 per 1000.)

Death rate. The number of deaths occurring per unit of population during a specified period of time. The crude death rate is usually calculated by relating total deaths in a year to the total mid-year population. (Crude death rate in England and Wales in 1985 was 12 per 1000.)

Fertility rate. The number of live births occurring in a year related to the number of women in the population of child-bearing age, usually 15–44 years. (Fertility rate in England and Wales in 1985 was 61 per 1000.)

Incidence rate. The number of events, such as onset of symptoms or diagnosis, related to the size of the population and a specified time.

Prevalence rate. The number of people with a condition, such as a symptom or pathological lesion, at any one time related to the size of the population.

Proportional mortality and morbidity rates. These express the number of cases of a disease as a proportion of cases of all kinds treated or dying in the same hospital, clinic or area. Proportional rates have been widely used in cancer epidemiology in non-industrialized countries, where the number of cases of one form of cancer is expressed as a proportion of the number of cases of all forms of cancer attending the same hospital. This method of expressing disease frequency is liable to errors, for the frequency of a disease may appear to rise or fall solely because of changes in the frequency of others. Generally, proportional rates should be used only in circumstances where population data are unavailable.

Special incidence rates. These include:

1. *Admission rates.* The number of admissions to hospital per unit of population during a specified period of time. These share with attack rates and consultation rates (see below) the characteristic of being derived from numbers of episodes and not numbers of persons.

2. *Attack rates.* The number of episodes of a disease in relation to the size of the population at risk and a specified period of time.

3. *Consultation rate.* The number of general practitioner consultations for a condition in relation to the size of the practice list and a specified period of time.

Special mortality rates. These include:

1. *Case fatality ratio.* The proportion of episodes of disease that end fatally.

2. *Infant mortality rates.* The number of infants (children under the age of 1 year) who die during a stated year per 1000 live births occurring in the same year. (The infant mortality rate in England and Wales in 1985 was 9 per 1000 live births.)

3. *Neonatal mortality rates.* The number of children who die in the neonatal period (up to 28 days after birth) during a stated year

per 1000 live births occurring in the same year. (The neonatal mortality rate in England and Wales in 1985 was 5 per 1000 live births.)

4. *Perinatal mortality rates*. The number of stillbirths plus the number of deaths in the first 7 days after birth during a stated year per 1000 total births (live births plus stillbirths). It is known that a proportion of the deaths that occur within a few days after birth are incorrectly registered as stillbirths, thereby inflating the stillbirth rate and lowering the neonatal mortality rate. The perinatal mortality rate, being a combination of late fetal and early neonatal deaths, is not influenced by this error. Furthermore, the two types of death have certain common causes, for example toxaemia and birth trauma. (The perinatal mortality rate in England and Wales in 1985 was 10 per 1000 births.)

5. *Postneonatal mortality rates*. The number of infant deaths after the first 28 days of life during a stated year per 1000 live births occurring in the same year. (The postneonatal mortality rate in England and Wales in 1985 was 4 per 1000 live births.)

6. *Stillbirth rates*. The number of stillbirths (intra-uterine deaths after the 28th week of pregnancy) occurring during 1 year in every 1000 total births. (The stillbirth rate in England and Wales during 1985 was 6 per 1000 total births)

Index

Response rate in surveys, 44
Retrolental fibroplasia, 108
Ringworm, hazards of irradiation, 81
Risk
  attributable, 80, 95–96
  relative, 80, 96

Sample, recruitment of, 42–44
Sample size, 41–42
Sampling, 42–44
Scatter diagrams, 91–92
Schizophrenia, 66
Screening, 125–134
Seasonal variations, 60–62, 72–73
Secular trends, 6–7, 57–59, 74–77
Semelweiss, 108
Sensitivity of test, 36–37, 130
Sex ratios, 63–64
Sickness absence, 9–10, 24, 61
Significance testing, 92–93, 107
Smoking
  and birth weight, 102
  and lung cancer, 97,
  trials of cessation, 102
Snow, John, 100, 135
Social class, definitions of, 64
Social drift, 66
Social security statistics, 24
Socio-economic status and disease, 8,
  64–65
Space-time clustering, 76–77
Specificity of test, 36–37, 130
Standard error, 41–42
Standardisation of rates, 54–57

Standardised mortality ratio, 54
Stillbirths, 57, 159
Surveillance, 146
Surveys, 29–48
  clinical, 29, 113–116
  cross-sectional, 38–46
  longitudinal, 46–48
  occupational, 83, 48
  prospective, 80
  record design in, 45–46, 117
  retrospective, 80
Survival rates, 119–121

Time trends, 6–7, 57–62, 74–77
Thyrotoxicosis, 60–61
Tonsillectomy, 148
Toxic allergic syndrome, 138
Trials, randomised controlled,
  104–107, 129, 152, 153
Typhoid, 99

Utilisation of services, 150

Validity of measurements, 35–37,
  130–131
Variation
  observer, 30–35
  subject (biological), 34
Volunteers, use in surveys, 42–43

Whooping cough, 21–22, 103
Wilson's disease, 133